CW00894149

# OPTIMIZED UNDER 35

## HOW TO BOOST TESTOSTERONE, INCREASE YOUR SEX DRIVE, AND ACHIEVE INCREDIBLE HEALTH

DANIEL KELLY

Optimized Under 35: How to Boost Testosterone, Increase Your Sex Drive, and Achieve Incredible Health

Copyright © 2019 by Daniel Kelly

All Rights Reserved. No part of this book or any of its contents may be reproduced, copied, modified, distributed, stored, transmitted in any form or by any means, or adapted without the prior written consent of the authors and publisher.

This book is not intended as a substitute for the medical advice of physicians. The reader should regularly consult a physician in matters relating to his/her health and particularly with respect to any symptoms that may require diagnosis or medical attention.

Publishing services provided by 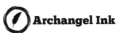 Archangel Ink

ISBN-13: 978-1-7903-8115-9

# IN MEMORY OF DR. JOHN CRISLER

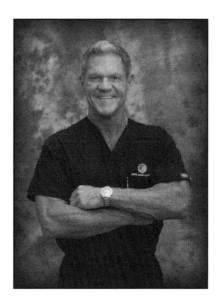

I would like to dedicate this book to the memory of Dr. John Crisler, who sadly passed away before this book was published in January 2019.

Dr. Crisler was a legend and pioneer in the hormone optimization field. He began prescribing testosterone replacement therapy in the early 2000s, when TRT was still very much a taboo, and his work help established the now mainstream practice.

Dr. Crisler believed TRT could help men and was willing to blaze a new trail in medicine, an industry that doesn't always reward innovation. I admired him for his outspoken views and courage of conviction. He ruffled some feathers in the process, but that's what made him even more likeable.

Before I started testosterone replacement therapy, I read Dr. Crisler's book back to back several times. He was instrumental in my decision to undergo treatment. It was reassuring to know that such an accomplished man and leading doctor, who was also in great physical shape, had also chosen to undergo TRT.

Dr Crisler was a leader in his field because he always remembered that people become doctors to serve others, and he lived this service in everything he did.

Dr. Crisler was generous with his time and advice with everyone, including me. When I was a nobody, hoping to get interviews with leading figures for this book, he was gracious with his time. He sat down and answered my questions and asked for nothing in return. He was a hero of mine, and he was willing to be interviewed for this book.

During the interview, I was in awe of his knowledge and insight. Indeed, it is one of the best in the book. Not only that; I was taken aback by his friendly demeanor and modesty.

Dr. Crisler was a remarkable man and a true visionary that touched and changed the lives of countless men and women. I would not have been able to write this book without his courage to lead the way when no one else would or could.

I had hoped to meet John in the near future and personally thank him and give him a copy of my own book. It breaks my heart and brings tears to my eyes knowing that I will never meet John in person.

Thank you for everything you did John. You won't be forgotten.

England, January 2019

# CONTENTS

# FOREWORD BY JAY CAMPBELL

A little over five years ago, Daniel Kelly wrote me an email out of the blue after listening to a podcast I did with Mike Cernovich. Little did I know that five years later he would be an empowered thought leader on a mission to teach young men about the benefits of therapeutic testosterone for lifelong health and happiness.

It gives me a great sense of enjoyment to see him flourish after many late-night Zoom video calls and WhatsApp conversations from across the pond. I remember how fearful he was contemplating the use of therapeutic testosterone because there were so few doctors in the UK even capable of providing him the quality of care he deserved. I had to back him off the ledge many times due to the soul-crushing indecisiveness that suboptimal levels of testosterone cause.

Fast-forward to today. Daniel's tweets and social media posts are erudite and inspiring for so many young men lost in a world of soy and suboptimal hormones. With his new book, *Optimized Under 35,* Daniel has become one of the leading voices in the realm of optimization in the international community. In this book, Daniel offers his unique perspective as a young man who optimized his hormones at an age when few men even understand they have a problem.

You should be incredibly excited! Right now you're holding a book with the power to revolutionize the medical landscape and radically improve your day-to-day life. It is one of the first to recognize the horrific societal epidemic of suboptimal hormones and how they wreak havoc on the lives of young men. This epidemic is ongoing and currently unrecognized by modern medicine (aka the sick care system). Not only is there a lack of recognition by the scientific community, there is an even greater lack of understanding by the medical community (doctors) to identify, treat, and solve the issue.

But fear not, Daniel's book IS your blueprint to cutting through the testosterone booster nonsense while informing you every step of the way. It will guide you through the science on utilizing therapeutic testosterone to maximize your life from every conceivable angle. While this book is aimed at men age 18–35, the truth is that men of any age will get something out of it.

Daniel's approach will teach you how to be more assertive in your workplace and more powerful around women. You'll grow stronger, leaner, and more muscular from your training. Ultimately, you'll become spiritually fit from all the internal work instruction he provides.

Take full control of your life by reading and implementing the strategies he offers you.

–Jay Campbell
TRT Expert at totrevolution.com

# IMPORTANT: YOUR FREE BONUS

As a thank you for purchasing this book, I'd like to give you a free bonus:

**10 Powerful Ways to Cultivate Your Masculine Energy**

This e-book builds on many of the topics we'll cover here in *Optimized Under 35*, and I'm confident you'll enjoy it.

You can get your free bonus by going to the following link: www.optimizedarmy.com/masculine-energy

Signing up means you'll be notified of book releases and receive regular content on becoming the CEO of your health. You'll also be first in line for exclusive deals on anything I put out.

Immediately after signing up you'll be sent an email with access to the bonus.

Go grab it now!

–Daniel Kelly

# ACKNOWLEDGMENTS

The idea of a self-made man is a fallacy. The reality is, no one gets where they are without help from others. I've always felt it's important to acknowledge the people in my life who have helped me along my personal journey. I want to take the opportunity here to thank the people who helped make this book a reality.

First off, I want to thank my coach and mentor, Kirsty Hanly, who helped me overcome my resistance to writing this book. It would never have made it to print if she hadn't shown me its importance.

Next, I want to thank Jay Campbell for being an exceptional friend and mentor over the years, and for his guidance when I first began testosterone replacement therapy. Without him, I probably would never have started therapy in the first place.

I want to thank Dominik Grueneberg for being an incredibly supportive friend. He gave me honest and insightful feedback and constant encouragement as I wrote this book.

Thanks to Tony Monticone, who was always in my corner as I wrote this book and got my business off the ground. He believed in me when others doubted me, and even when I doubted myself.

Mike Kocsis was instrumental in my ability to write this book because he so generously passed on his knowledge of testosterone replacement therapy. His wisdom and experience are unparalleled in this field.

I would also like to thank Paul Burgess for his mentorship, particularly in teaching me to take a holistic view of health instead of a one-track view.

Also, thanks to Sam Mitchell and Jason Grey for taking the time out of their busy schedules to read the book and provide detailed feedback.

In addition, I would like to thank Austin Gunter for his brilliant editorial oversight, giving me the honest feedback I needed.

# INTRODUCTION

# MY JOURNEY TO OPTIMIZED HEALTH

I've been fascinated by health and fitness from the time I was a child. Simply being outdoors—exercising and playing sports—was more than enough. And I continued to play sports throughout school and college, from soccer to rugby to martial arts. Even though I wasn't especially gifted, I was an athlete at heart.

A lifelong passion was sparked at the age of 21 when I took up weight training. I vividly remember going to the gym with my friend, who showed me some basic exercises. At first I had no clue how to do them properly, but I loved pushing my mind and body beyond their limits. Indeed, I've always had a deep-seated desire to be the best version of myself, and it found expression through weight training.

After spending a few months in the gym, I noticed some serious changes in my body. Not only did I gain muscle, but I noticed girls checking me out more. My confidence soared, and I saw this reflected in how people responded to me. Even at this early stage, it was apparent to me that physical health had the power to not only change the way I looked and felt, but to change my entire life.

## BREAKING BAD HABITS

Despite seeing positive changes in my body composition and my life in general, I knew there was still room for improvement. For starters, my diet was subpar. I didn't know much about nutrition, but I was fortunate to have a fast metabolism. I could eat pretty much whatever I wanted, although I still tried to be selective. The problem was, I just didn't know what the right foods were, and I had no idea how important nutrition was to building muscle, let alone knowing about macro or micronutrients.

I took it upon myself to learn as much as I could about nutrition, and specifically how it related to building a great physique. Trying to put the pieces of the puzzle together, I spent hours trawling the Internet and experimenting with every type of diet out there—from intermittent fasting to carb cycling to paleo. I learned many key lessons during those years of trial and error. I don't regret the things I tried because each experiment got me a step closer to finding what worked and what didn't.

Even though I spent much time honing my diet and physique, I still refused to acknowledge the elephant in the room: while I was focused on the small aspect of lifting weights and developing proper nutrition, other areas of my lifestyle were out of balance. In my early twenties I smoked, drank way too much alcohol, and even took drugs occasionally. Yet, I thought I was healthy because I lifted weights and ate clean. Moreover, I only smoked when I drank, so I wasn't a "real" smoker, right? And binge drinking only on the weekend meant I wasn't abusing my body with alcohol, right? Wrong!

Because I was deep inside the hard-living London bubble at the time, the fact I was a major hypocrite didn't occur to me. Most of the people I associated with did the same thing. A "work hard, play harder" mentality was ingrained in the culture. However, deep down I knew I needed to change—I just didn't know how.

## GIVING UP THE GHOST

In dramatic transformations, there is usually a tipping point that acts as a catalyst for a breakthrough. Mine came one Saturday morning as I lay motionless on the couch in my apartment. My head was pounding, and my stomach felt like a lead balloon; I reeked of smoke and was incapacitated from a terrible hangover. My brain wouldn't function, so I vegetated to mind-numbing daytime TV, and taking regular trips to the bathroom to vomit the contents of my stomach into the toilet.

Everyone who has had a hangover has uttered the words, "I'm never drinking again!" But I knew this time was different. I'd had enough. I was sick of spending my weekends feeling like this and paying the price for my hedonism. Here I was, training hard and eating right all week only to throw it all away at the weekend. In an attempt to cut down my drinking, I tried to limit the number of drinks I had when I went out. Little did I know my plan was doomed from the start. Friday night rolled around, and I was determined to go to the bar, hang out with my friends, and end the night at one or two drinks. But this happened rarely, if *ever*. Before I knew it, I was waking up in my bed the next day fully clothed, wondering what the hell happened.

It felt like I was fighting a losing battle with alcohol. And what's more, I hadn't even addressed the smoking! So I decided to change tack; I set my sights on giving up cigarettes. One day I went to see the doctor to ask about using nicotine patches—I figured they would help kill my craving for cigarettes. Fortunately, the doctor agreed to help me but not in the way I expected. He refused to give me nicotine patches, telling me to go cold turkey on cigarettes instead.

I was indignant. How on earth was I going to manage that? The cravings were almost unbearable when I drank alcohol. Then he told me something I'll never forget, "You need to give up cigarettes using your willpower because you will learn a lot about yourself in the process. If alcohol gives you cravings, then stop drinking alcohol until it goes away." Bizarre as it sounds, this solution had never occurred to me. Give up alcohol altogether? *Only zealots and health freaks do that*, I mused. But, thankfully, I was willing to try it because my desire to change had become so strong.

After failing to quit alcohol, I resolved not to make the same mistake with cigarettes. If I was going to succeed, I knew I had to change the way I saw this habit. Instead of seeing cigarettes as the problem, I chose to focus on the cues or triggers that enabled the habit in the first place. For instance, going to bars, drinking alcohol, and being around people who smoked triggered my cravings to smoke. So I reasoned that if I removed them from the equation, I would be able to kick the cravings.

In the beginning, I felt like a social outcast and was worried I was missing out (FOMO!) while my friends were having fun. However, after a few weeks, the cravings completely disappeared, and I managed to quit cigarettes for good. It seems the wily old doctor knew a thing or two after all. Best of all, this experience showed me alcohol had no place in my life. The doctor told me that cigarettes only took away and didn't add anything to my life. I concluded it was the same with alcohol; I was not a slave to societal norms—I was free to make my own choices.

Finally, I managed to overcome my demons; I was leading the healthy lifestyle I had always aspired to, a lifestyle I **would not compromise for anyone**. By conventional standards, I followed a strict diet, though I still allowed myself to indulge and enjoy food. The difference was I no longer had anything holding me back! Now I could focus on getting stronger and fitter without feeling like I was taking two steps back every weekend.

## A VERDICT OF LOW TESTOSTERONE

Two years after kicking my bad habits to the curb, I was going strong. Then I heard a podcast where Mike Cernovich and Jay Campbell discussed testosterone replacement therapy, underlining the importance of having regular blood work done from an early age. The idea was: getting regular blood work allows you to collect data on your health so you can anticipate and deal with any issues that arise instead of being blindsided by them. Instinctively, I knew this was something I wanted to do in my journey to optimize my health.

So in 2014 I took my first testosterone test at the age of 27. I didn't have any symptoms of low testosterone, so I figured everything would be fine. The result revealed I had serum testosterone of 540 ng/dL (19 nmol/L). At the time, I thought this was okay because it appeared to be in the mid-range of normal. In reality, however, it was in the lower quartile of normal. Looking back now, I can see the writing was already on the wall.

After the serious changes I'd made in my life, things were going well as I entered my late twenties. Although I no longer gained muscle the way I had when I first began training, my progress in the gym was steady and consistent—until I reached the age of 28. Over the course of only one year, I noticed I struggled to make any real gains in strength or size and was unable to lose body fat, despite the fact I was training harder than ever.

I couldn't figure out what the issue was. My diet was on point, I didn't drink or smoke, I slept enough, and I minimized stress in my life. Ultimately, I concluded I had reached the mythical "genetic ceiling" and maxed out my gains at the ripe old age of 28! Was it going to be like this for the rest of my life—training hard in the gym for mediocre to nonexistent results? This was the first sign something was wrong.

A year after taking my first testosterone test, I went for my self-imposed yearly checkup. It was supposed to be routine; I wasn't prepared for what happened next. All the markers in my blood panel appeared to be perfectly normal—until I got to testosterone.

I had a serum testosterone level of 230 ng/dL (8 nmol/L). This was the same testosterone level as an 80-year-old man. Except I was 28! I was dumbstruck. It felt like someone had punched me in the stomach, and it took me several days to get over the shock. How could my testosterone be so low when I lived such a healthy lifestyle?

Once I got myself together, I decided to take another blood test to rule out any anomalies. The second test measured my serum testosterone at 345 ng/dL (12 nmol/L). It was marginally better than my previous test, but it was certainly not optimal for a man my age. I was basically running on empty! Truth be told, I was distraught and in complete disarray. I had no idea why this was happening to me.

Despite my anguish, the one thing these tests gave me was clarity. Suddenly, so many things in my life made sense. Anxiety had been a thorn in my side for some time, and I suffered from regular panic attacks. I used to get chest pains and convinced myself I was having a heart attack. I had even gone to the hospital emergency room on several occasions, though nothing was ever found to be wrong.

Eventually, I managed to get the panic attacks under control with the help of a psychiatrist. But the anxiety never really disappeared; it persisted in the form of daily, grinding anxiety. My stomach was always in knots, and I worried endlessly over the most trivial things. However, that was the least of my problems. To add to my despair, my sex drive had fallen off a cliff. I would go weeks without feeling any sort of sexual desire. It even got to the point where sex felt like a chore! Something that was once so enjoyable now held no interest. This was bizarre indeed.

Before I understood my testosterone levels, I figured I was just going through a difficult time, hoping it would eventually sort itself out. It never did. On the outside, I tried to pretend everything was okay. But in reality, I felt empty and miserable inside. Some days I didn't want to get out of bed. I preferred to wallow in my own pity. And I became so apathetic toward life, it no longer mattered whether I lived or died.

After the blood test, I had a revelation: I had been suffering the hallmark symptoms of low testosterone. My progress in the gym had ground to a halt—not because I had maxed out my genetic potential, **but because I had no testosterone to build any muscle**. The anxiety, low sex drive, and depression weren't personal issues; they **were a consequence of low testosterone**.

You may ask how I didn't recognize the symptoms of low testosterone, especially since I knew what they were. Here's the thing: I was convinced low testosterone couldn't possibly affect me at such a young age, especially because I led a healthy lifestyle. What's more, I was so focused on getting results in the gym that I failed to see my whole life was unraveling. The symptoms of low testosterone don't come on suddenly and all at once—they gradually creep up on you like a thief in the night. Eventually, you forget what it's like to live without these symptoms and you accept them as normal. It's a strange kind of Stockholm syndrome. As a result, I had unwittingly incorporated anxiety, depression, a low sex drive, and poor performance in the gym as part of my identity.

Nevertheless, I knew deep down this was not who I really was. Something inside of me refused to accept it. This was no way to live as a man. It was clear to me that my issue was medical, and not psychological or lifestyle-related. So I decided to take action.

## GETTING A PRESCRIPTION FOR TESTOSTERONE

I knew that if I were to undergo testosterone replacement therapy, I would be on medication for the rest of my life. This thought terrified me, but I couldn't go on living this way. Consequently, I immersed myself in research, read everything there was to read on testosterone, and spent countless hours scouring online medical journals and scientific studies.

The quest to find a qualified and *competent* doctor was not easy. Then, as today, there were few doctors in the UK willing to treat young men with testosterone replacement therapy. After searching all corners of the Internet, I finally found a doctor who might treat me.

I arrived at the appointment armed with research to handle any objections he might have to treating me. I even took him a copy of Jay Campbell's *The Definitive Testosterone Replacement Therapy MANual!* Thankfully, the doctor was very open to treating me. He did a painstaking analysis of my blood tests and symptoms, and he answered my concerns.

This was not what I'd expected. It was a two-way conversation based on mutual respect, instead of a one-way monologue in which the doctor dictated the terms. And I felt he genuinely cared about what I wanted. Taken aback, I asked him about this open approach; it was something I had seldom witnessed. He told me, "In over 20 years of prescribing hormones, I've learned to listen to the patient because they are the ones who live in their body, not me."

We agreed to start me out on clomiphene (Clomid) to address the low testosterone. Clomid simultaneously helps maintain fertility and raise testosterone. Given my age and the fact I wanted to father children in the future, this was a sensible first step. After talking with other men who were TRT patients, though, I felt testosterone would be preferable to Clomid. This is because several men told me they felt subpar on Clomid and felt bloated and moody, whereas the majority waxed lyrical about testosterone. After discussing this with the doctor, we decided I would go on injectable testosterone.

## OVERCOMING RESISTANCE TO CHANGE

In January 2016 I received my prescription from the doctor and got the medication from the pharmacy. It would be 200 mg of Sustanon a week, split into two injections. So here I was on the verge of change. I had done my research and finally had my prescription. Mission accomplished, right? Well, even though I knew testosterone would bring about positive change to my life, I was still scared SHITLESS.

All the worst-case scenarios played over and over in my head. What if it didn't work out? What the FUCK was I doing? Had I really thought this through?

In hindsight, I see these fears had no basis in reality. But the prospect of undergoing TRT was daunting, and I allowed my fears to get the better of me. Several weeks passed, and I did nothing. I couldn't summon up the courage to inject, so I kept putting it off. Fortunately, my good friend Jay Campbell saw through my charade. He told me in no uncertain terms to "stop being a pussy and INJECT." It was tough love, but it was exactly what I needed, and it woke me from my stupor.

As a side note, this experience underlined to me that every man needs a real friend in his life to tell him the truth. Even if the truth hurts at first. And while I'm not religious, Jesus said it right: "Then you will know the truth, and the truth will set you free" (John 8:32, NIV).

I wish I could tell you I had an iron will and taking testosterone didn't faze me. But it wasn't like that. In fact, I had to get my roommate to do the first injections for me. However, after a few injections I realized they were no big deal, and not the monster I made them out to be. After a month I didn't even think about it; it was like brushing my teeth.

Ultimately, the biggest battle was overcoming my own resistance to change, which is really a metaphor for life. My fear about taking testosterone didn't immediately subside. A few weeks after I started treatment, a friend came over to visit me. We had the usual chitchat, and then he asked how my treatment was going, at which point I broke down in tears in front of him. I felt ashamed and embarrassed that I allowed my emotions to get the better of me, especially in front of someone. But I couldn't help it. All of the pressure and pent-up emotion I'd felt over this just came out. I told him that I still worried whether I was making the right choice. However, a month later, the testosterone began to kick in, and my decision to do it was validated.

## HOW TESTOSTERONE TRANSFORMED MY LIFE

In early 2016, after overcoming my doubts and insecurities, I began to experience a huge shift in the way I looked, felt, and perceived the world. The testosterone was starting to work its magic. My libido came roaring back to life; I reveled once more in the joy of physical intimacy and female companionship. The ridiculous inadequacies I felt about myself and my self-consciousness around women faded. It wasn't that I became a sex maniac, lusting after every woman I saw; testosterone simply revitalized my sexual appetite and restored healthy balance.

The constant, daily anxiety was replaced by a steadfast calmness. Thoughts no longer swirled around in my head like violent waves in a storm, my mind no longer succumbed to panic and fear, and my body no longer convulsed with tension.

Prior to testosterone therapy, concentration was a huge problem for me; I struggled to focus on tasks for long periods. But after testosterone, the shroud of darkness that enveloped my mind was finally lifted. No more brain fog. My thinking became clearer and sharper, and I felt I had complete dominion over my mind, where before it felt like I had minimal control. Decision-making was better; I no longer agonized over things, and I made up my mind quickly.

I also saw significant improvement in the gym. My strength went up, and my stamina increased tenfold. Where before I was sore for days after a punishing workout, the soreness was almost nonexistent, and I could train more intensely. After just six months of intense training, I put on over 10 pounds, nearly all of which was lean muscle.

However, it wasn't just me who saw changes; other people noticed too. People responded to me differently. The confidence I felt was reflected in their positive attitude toward me. Hormone optimization helped me recognize something I always knew but rarely acknowledged: Your external reality is merely a reflection of your internal reality. They are not separate. They are one and the same.

Without testosterone, I would not be half the man I am today. Words cannot accurately describe the mental and physical metamorphosis I underwent. Testosterone helped me go from an unconfident, anxious, depressed shell of a man to a confident, assertive, and positive individual.

Why can't this be the same for you? Looking back, I was very fortunate to see some of the benefits of testosterone so quickly. Namely, improved libido, focus, and concentration. But it's important to note that I dedicated years to learning about proper nutrition, exercise, and lifestyle optimization, incorporating them all into my daily life. And, as you saw earlier, this wasn't an overnight process.

Like a plant that grows when given adequate sunlight, water, and nutrients, I created the right environment for testosterone to thrive. It felt like everything I did up until then had prepared me for this moment. As a result, once hormonal balance was restored, my life took off in dramatic fashion. **Testosterone was the catalyst for change, *not* the change itself.** The picture below on the left is me before I started TRT. The look on my face says it all; I was unsure, lacking self-confidence and afraid. And there was belly fat around my stomach that I just couldn't get rid of. The second picture on the right is me after being on testosterone for six months. I look much more confident and assured. But not only that, my physique has changed in dramatic fashion; I appear more defined and muscular. This is the power of hormonal balance.

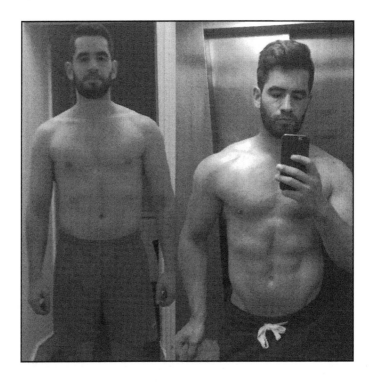

## THIS BOOK IS ABOUT YOU

Thankfully, I had friends who were on testosterone to guide and support me through this process. Still, that doesn't remove the fear and trepidation you experience about undergoing a lifelong treatment. In the end, you are the one who has to run the gauntlet and overcome your own obstacles to optimal health. And you are the one who must face down any psychological demons you have around therapy at such a young age.

That's why I've written this book. I want to show other young men what is possible with testosterone optimization.

Telling my personal story here isn't to show you how great I am. It's to show you where I came from and how I got here. Because if I can do it, so can you. **This book is about you, not me.**

# CHAPTER 1

# THE 21ˢᵀ CENTURY MALE AND DECLINE OF MASCULINITY

The 21ˢᵗ century male has become a maligned figure. The movement to empower women has swung the pendulum too far, so much so that men feel they've been left by the wayside. The dark side of feminism has spawned man-haters, and patriarchy is blamed for every societal ill.

In many ways, modern man has become superfluous to society's needs. In the name of empowerment, women are now expected to be independent of men. As more women provide for themselves, the man no longer needs to be the breadwinner. And oftentimes, the government acts as a surrogate father to a family.

However, when a man does show up, speak out, and stand his ground, he becomes an easy target for those looking to lay blame. These days, strong male role models are hard to find. Being a man in the traditional sense of the word is taboo, and masculinity is discouraged and shunned. In this chapter, we will explore the role culture has had on masculinity, and why it has become so maligned in today's society.

## THE NEW NORM FOR MEN

For many young men today, a low-energy, low libido, anxiety-ridden existence is the norm. And because they've always felt this way and have been surrounded by men in the same boat, they don't know there's an alternative. This negative feedback loop leads them to believe this is how it is to be a man. Nature has a purpose for everything, and men were not meant to retreat from life. We are wired to take action; we are meant to build businesses, invent things, and make positive contributions to society.

However, it appears many young men have checked out of society altogether. They live a vapid existence staying home and playing video games. They live in a dream world where virtual reality is the only reality, and the real world is merely an unwanted distraction from their virtual one. They would rather masturbate to women on a porn site than go out and talk to real women. Their communication skills are terrible because most of their interactions are via text messages and social media. When I was a kid, playing video games was just a pastime. For many kids today, playing video games is their entire existence, so we have a generation of young men who have turned into social recluses. This has serious ramifications for our society.

Fewer men in society means plummeting birth rates. Lower birth rates mean fewer young people arriving into the workforce to replace those retiring. The only possible outcome is societal decline and economic stagnation. History cautions us that empires rise and fall. In generations to come, people will look back at our own history to pinpoint exactly where it started.

If you want to see how social isolation affects society, look no further than Japan. Once admired by the rest of the world, Japan's economy became a basket case in the 1990s and has struggled to recover ever since. Japan has an aging population, its birth rates are declining, and 2016 marked a **117-year low** in fertility rates in Japan. How did this happen? While Japan's problems are complex and unique, one explanation could be the Japanese phenomenon known as *Hikikomori*. This is where people, mostly men, confine themselves to their homes for years, rarely leaving to go outside to interact with the outside world, resulting in what many call "the lost generation."[1]

## THE LOST GENERATION?

Another reason young men fail to form a strong masculine identity is they've never had a positive male role model. Oftentimes, fathers, browbeaten by society themselves, were poor role models who were either physically or emotionally absent. Relying on women and teachers to act as surrogate fathers for our boys is a failed experiment on a grand scale. Men need fathers in their lives to teach them how to be men. What's more, we can no longer treat boys as misbehaving girls, brainwashing them to deny their basic instincts—as if being a boy is somehow morally wrong.

Similarly, we have no rite of passage to mark the transition from adolescence into manhood. For instance, the Native Americans, Egyptians, and Vikings understood the need for men to have a rite of passage into manhood. It gave them a strong sense of identity and affirmed their place in society. When they demonstrated their worth as men, they would be treated as men by their peers. The ancients lived in an unforgiving world, where men needed to grow up quickly; failure to do so could mean the difference between life and death. War was always around the corner. Rites of passage weren't arbitrary rituals; they prepared men to become future leaders. Unfortunately, today we teach young men how to memorize elements of the periodic table instead of equipping them with the necessary skills to succeed in the world.

You don't need to lead a raiding party to make the transition into manhood. A modern rite of passage might be a father taking his son

---

1 William Kremer and Claudia Hammond, "Hikikomori: Why are so many Japanese men refusing to leave their rooms?" BBC News, July 5, 2013, http://www.bbc.com/news/magazine-23182523.

on a fishing or hunting trip, or simply giving him responsibilities around the house. Indeed, doing these things makes a boy feel like a man, and gives him a sense of pride in his masculine identity. Sadly, however, these things rarely happen today. This skewed identity and lack of role models has left men to figure things out for themselves. Now we have a generation of boys that never left adolescence and don't know their place in the world. So they do what boys do—they behave like boys.

The Sexual Revolution in the 1960s signaled the emancipation of women and more equality in society as a whole. However, gender equality has morphed into gender obscurity, blurring the lines between men and women. Young men are brainwashed with anti-male vitriol in educational institutions and taught that masculine behavior is wrong. "Toxic masculinity" and "patriarchy" are all too often held up as scapegoats for all society's ills.

As a result, many young men have become effeminate and soft—both mentally and physically. They would not be able to defend themselves or their families if it came to it. They don't say what they mean, nor do they have the courage and conviction to do so. Passive aggressive behavior is commonplace, and most men will cower if you look them in the eye. Being direct and honest in conversation is seen as offensive, as if speaking your mind is somehow threatening and malicious. Millennials are arguably one of the most socially engineered generations in history. Through social media, technology, and education, they've been conditioned to behave a certain way. I call this the Millennial Complex.

## THE MILLENNIAL COMPLEX

Reality has become totally distorted by social media. Sometimes this becomes so extreme that people think social media *is* reality. We think the highlight reel people post on social media is a true reflection of the lives they lead, and our self-worth is based on the amount of likes we get on an Instagram post. We think that racking up points on Call of Duty or spending time arguing on Reddit calling people "cucks" has genuine meaning.

All their lives, Millennials have been mollycoddled and told, "Be yourself! You're fine as you are!" And to a certain degree, I agree with this: it's important to be yourself. But you must be the most authentic version of yourself, the person you are in your heart. And sometimes it takes work to develop your God-given talent in order to realize your most authentic self. Sadly, many Millennials believe that "Be yourself" means you just have to show up and success is assured.

The whole "Be yourself" deceit also stems from a low sense of self-esteem and self-worth. When you have low self-worth, platitudes are easy to believe. Whereas someone with a strong sense of self-worth accepts themselves for who they are; they know "Be yourself!" is empty drivel that doesn't pay the bills or put food on the table.

Millennials believe just by virtue of showing up they will get what they want. Showered with gifts by well-meaning Baby Boomer parents from a young age, many Millennials have been conditioned to have everything they ever wanted—an iPad, a new car, etc. Loving parents want to pamper their children, providing them with the best life possible. But in doing so, they created a monster. Children who have everything handed to them don't appreciate the value of hard work or the resilience and determination required to achieve things when life gets tough.

As a result, Millennials often lack necessary humility, dismissing the experience of others because they already "know it all." This is reflected in the deep disdain many young people have for history and ancient wisdom. In fact, I can't believe how few young people today know about history—not because it's a fun subject, but as the saying goes, "Forget the lessons of history at your peril."

What this all leads to is a deep sense of entitlement. This entitlement was manifest in riots and violence throughout the United States during the summer of 2017. These events centered around [mainly young] people's discontent with the political system. Chaos and anarchy ensued; people were injured; buildings and vehicles were set ablaze. This was the response of a people who felt they had been wronged by the government and by society. They thought everything would be given to them, and when it wasn't, they pulled out the victim card. When they didn't get their way, they resorted to violence.

These are people who would rather wallow in self-pity than take responsibility for their lives. Everything is always someone else's fault or the government's fault. However, playing the blame game won't solve anyone's problems. Unfortunately, society only reinforces their lack of personal responsibility. Dr. Joe Dispenza explains how we often unwittingly become addicted to our emotions in his ground-breaking book, *Becoming Supernatural: How Common People Are Doing the Uncommon.*

For example, if anger, resentment, and frustration is all you've ever known, these emotions remain your default state. Even if Millennials like those I've described above want to get out of this cycle, the body accepts this state as the "normal" environment, activating genes and releasing chemicals to perpetuate this emotional state. Subsequently, these people perpetuate their state of learned helplessness, not knowing they were the cause of their own pain all along.

## THE KINGPIN MINDSET

In addition to the Millennial Complex, there is another attitude at work among young Millennials, which I call the "Kingpin Mindset." Kingpin is a Marvel character who started out life as a common thug in the Bronx. He eventually worked his way up through the ranks to become a crime boss. Above all, Kingpin is renowned for his lavish lifestyle and spending habits, including fancy suits, watches, and expensive cigars.

So what is the Kingpin Mindset? The Kingpin Mindset refers to young men who adopt an online persona that revolves around displays of wealth and success. They go on social media and post endless pictures of bottle parties, boutique hotels, expensive watches, high-performance cars, cigars, and models. Don't get me wrong, I have nothing against these things. But like Kingpin, these guys feel if they associate themselves with luxury and wealth, they will earn the respect and admiration of others. However, once you lift the veil, the lives these men lead are rarely like they portray on social media.

So the question becomes, why do they feel so compelled to portray their lives this way? There are complex reasons for this, but the bottom line is these men feel insecure and lack self-esteem, so they think associating themselves with a stereotype of success will give them acceptance. And because they don't have male role models in their lives, they haven't learned the value of developing their character. Now, bravado and boasting are part of being a young man. However, the advent of social media has taken these attributes to an unhealthy level. I don't hold anything against these guys. I actually think it's a sad indictment of society that men feel pressured to appear a certain way.

Their message is often positive and aspirational, and many times the story follows the archetype of the rags-to-riches story. So you can

27

see why these men might attract followers, because other guys want to achieve a similar transformation. However the problem is, they're also teaching young men to adopt the Kingpin Mindset and become dysfunctional like they are. The Internet is already full of inauthentic people; it doesn't need more people teaching impressionable, naïve young men to pursue an empty existence.

## TESTOSTERONE AND MASCULINITY: AN INSEPARABLE DUO

While we've seen there are many cultural factors that have characterized men's fall from grace, this is not all there is to it. In my opinion, this state of "learned helplessness" can be rectified in many young men by addressing their hormonal imbalances.

Where there is a decline in masculinity, you can guarantee there is also a decline in testosterone. You can't write a book on hormone optimization and testosterone without discussing masculinity; the two are inextricably linked. Blood levels of testosterone are literally what separate a male from a female at birth. After all, strong-willed men are not easy to tame and socially engineer, but weak and docile men are.

Unfortunately, because they don't know any different and because testosterone levels are in the gutter, effectively castrating their manhood, most men think this is normal. These same young men have never experienced optimal testosterone levels surging through their veins and the incredible confidence and steadfast resolve it provides in their daily life.

This "low-T reality" has infested many areas of society to the point that it's unacceptable to bring up traditional or conservative views in polite conversation. And if you don't agree with mainstream ideology, you're a "sexist pig" or whatever buzzword is fashionable today. But don't stop there; if you're a straight man, you had better check your privilege for showing an ounce of masculinity! Make no mistake, it's not "toxic masculinity" that's the problem. It's the toxic "progressive" ideology that hates anything masculine that poses a real threat to society.

Don't get me wrong: there is no doubt that masculine energy channeled the wrong way can be a negative and destructive force. We only have to look at the world's history of nonstop war and violence to see this. However, this shadow side of the male psyche is not the *only* side, as some would have you believe, nor is it true masculinity. True masculinity is something entirely different. It's what makes Navy SEALs endure months of grueling training to risk their lives on missions. It's what makes firemen scale ladders and go into blazing infernos to save lives. It's what makes a man get up every day to go to a job he doesn't like so he can put food on the table for his family. Among other things, true masculinity represents strength, integrity, and stability. These traits have served our ancestors for millennia, yet today they are shunned in favor of the progressive ideal of how a man "should be."

We have been sold the lie that *toxic masculinity* is at the heart of most of society's problems. When in reality, a severe *lack of masculinity* is one of society's biggest issues. When there is no masculinity in society, there is no order. And where there is no order, there is chaos.

Is it any wonder our society is in disarray when testosterone levels are at an all-time low? The simple truth is: When men don't have adequate levels of testosterone, they cease to function properly. And when men don't function properly, society breaks down. Today, we have an entire generation of young men who have likely NEVER experienced optimal levels of testosterone. They never went through the "raging hormones" stage as teenagers, where they thought about sex 24/7, wanted to play sports, were driven to compete with other men, or just felt compelled to do things that men do. Essentially, they have no idea what it means to be a man because their testosterone levels were so low to begin with.

If we want to go about rectifying the shameful loss of the masculine presence in our society, we have to start with restoring optimal hormonal balance. Because without your hormones in balance, your health declines. Proper health is the foundation on which your life is built. Without it, you have nothing. Men need to get back to basics and understand what's happening to them from the inside out.

# CHAPTER 2

# WHY HORMONAL BALANCE MATTERS TO YOU

L ooking after your health today is not like it was 50 years ago. Previous generations ate less food, and most of it was high-quality. They led more active lives, and the pollution in the environment from chemicals and human consumption was minimal. Essentially, their lifestyles were conducive to good health. Subsequently, they could remain in reasonable health for most of their lives without too much effort. They didn't have to work at being healthy—it was a way of life.

By comparison, today we eat mainly processed foods and genetically modified garbage. Food that was standard fare to our predecessors is now called "organic." Today's food lacks vital nutrients because it's sprayed with pesticides, pumped full of preservatives, and engineered to last forever on store shelves. Is it any wonder it bears zero resemblance to food of the past? Environmental pollution is rampant, and our bodies are exposed to all types of harmful toxins every day, especially endocrine disrupting chemicals (EDCs).

To put this in perspective, between 1960 and 2002, the weight of the average American male went from 166 pounds to 191 pounds![2] This comes as no surprise when we learn that in 2010 the average American consumed 2,481 calories a day—a 23% increase from 1970. And most of those calories come from grains and fat, particularly

---

2   Live Science, "Four-Decade Study: Americans Taller, Fatter," October 27, 2004, https://www.livescience.com/49-decade-study-americans-taller-fatter.html.

vegetable oils like soybean or canola. As we'll see later in this book, these substances are like kryptonite to your testosterone.

Cells in the human body communicate with each other through molecular messengers known as hormones. And the endocrine system acts as the manager for these hormones. Basically, the endocrine system is defined as any cell or organ in the body that produces and responds to hormones.[3] Hormones are responsible for regulating many of the body's functions, including growth, metabolism, and reproduction.[4]

The human endocrine system secretes some 50 different hormones. But why are hormones so important? Because they are the backbone of your health. And if you want to lead a life of health and vitality in today's world, you need to look after them. Don't worry; it's not important to understand them all. Focusing primarily on testosterone, which this book guides you to do, will create a domino effect. It alone has the power to initiate dramatic and positive change in your life.

## TESTOSTERONE: THE TIDE THAT LIFTS ALL THE SHIPS IN THE HARBOR

In men, testosterone is a hormone produced by the testes and is typically associated with increased vigor, virility, and strength. However, its role is multifaceted. It is needed to maintain androgenic (male) sex characteristics such as facial hair, a deep voice, sperm

---

3   George P Chrousos, "Organization and Integration of the Endocrine System," *Sleep Med Clin*, 2007 Jun, 2(2): 125–145, doi: 10.1016/j.jsmc.2007.04.004.

4   Hiller-Sturmhöfel, Bartke A, "The endocrine system: an overview," *Alcohol Health Res World*, 1998, 22(3): 153–64.

production, and muscle mass.[5] It has stimulatory effects on bones, libido, mood, cognition centers in the brain, and erectile strength. And it is also known to have a positive impact on metabolic rate, lipids (e.g., cholesterol), and inflammation.[6,7]

As you can see, testosterone influences all aspects of your health—mental, physical, and emotional. It's the centerpiece of your health. You will be a stronger, more confident, more positive, and overall more balanced individual with optimal testosterone levels. In fact, there is a direct correlation between your testosterone levels and your quality of life.

It's time for you to take your health seriously. Given testosterone is so crucial to a man's health, having a vague idea about it will no longer cut it. Your grandfather didn't have to worry about it and never took a testosterone test. You, on the other hand, do not possess such a luxury. By choosing to be part of modern life, you subject your body to a plethora of testosterone-lowering chemicals. So unless you live in a cave, knowing how to combat this onslaught and how to optimize your testosterone is no longer optional. It is ESSENTIAL.

5    "Peeyush Kumar, Nitish Kumar, Devendra Singh Thakur, and Ajay Patidar, "Male hypogonadism: Symptoms and treatment,"J Adv Pharm Technol Re, 2010 Jul-Sep; 1(3): 297–301.

6    Stella Vodo, Nicoletta Bechi, Anna Petroni, Carolina Muscoli, and Anna Maria Aloisi, "Testosterone-Induced Effects on Lipids and Inflammation," Mediators Inflamm, 2013: 183041.

7    Jerald Bain, "The many faces of testosterone," Clin Interv Aging, 2007 Dec, 2(4): 567–576.

# HOW IS TESTOSTERONE MADE?

Testosterone production begins in the brain with the hypothalamus and pituitary gland. The hypothalamus is found at the base of the brain and constitutes 2% of total brain mass.[8] It is one of the master controllers of your body. Among other things, it is responsible for maintaining homeostasis and works in tandem with the pituitary gland to secrete hormones.[9] In order to stimulate testosterone production, a series of interactions take place between the hypothalamus and pituitary gland; this process is known as the hypothalamic-pituitary-testicular axis (HPTA).

The process begins when the hypothalamus detects the body needs testosterone. It responds by secreting gonadotropin-releasing-hormone (GnRH). This signal then goes to the pituitary gland, which causes it to secrete both follicle stimulating hormone (FSH) and luteinizing hormone (LH). FSH is responsible for stimulating sperm production, while LH stimulates Leydig cells in the testes to produce testosterone. The Leydig cells take cholesterol from the bloodstream and convert it into pregnenolone, which is then converted into testosterone.[10] More than 95% of testosterone is produced from the Leydig cells in the testes, and a small amount is produced from the conversion of adrenal androgens.[11]

---

8   Ronald M Lechan, M.D., Ph.D. and Roberto Toni, M.D., Ph.D., "Functional Anatomy of the Hypothalamus and Pituitary," MDText.com, Inc.; 2000–.

9   Jakob Biran, Maayan Tahor, Einav Wircer, and Gil Levkowitz, "Role of developmental factors in hypothalamic function," published online 2015 Apr 21, doi: 10.3389/fnana.2015.00047.

10   K. Svechnikov, G. Izzo, L. Landreh, J. Weisser, and O. Söder, "Endocrine Disruptors and Leydig Cell Function," *J Biomed Biotechnol*, 2010: 684504, published online 2010 Aug 25, doi: 10.1155/2010/684504.

11   Megan Crawford and Laurence Kennedy, "Testosterone replacement therapy: role of pituitary and thyroid in diagnosis and treatment," *Transl Androl Urol*, 2016 Dec, 5(6): 850–858, doi: 10.21037/tau.2016.09.01.

Once testosterone is synthesized, it is released into the bloodstream for use by the body. The majority of the testosterone becomes bound to albumin and sex hormone binding globulin (SHBG). These carrier proteins are responsible for regulating concentrations of sex hormones in the blood.[12] In adult males, approximately 50% of testosterone is bound to albumin, 44% to SHBG, and 2–3% is unbound.[13] This remaining unbound testosterone is known as free testosterone.

Once the hypothalamus detects sufficient levels of testosterone in the blood, it sends a signal to the pituitary gland to cease production of LH. When the hypothalamus detects the need for more testosterone, the whole process starts again. This is known as the HPTA negative feedback loop, seen in the diagram below. It's long been thought testosterone is the key component in the HPTA negative feedback loop. However, there is also evidence in the literature to suggest estradiol (a form of estrogen) may actually be the prime regulator of gonadotropin levels (i.e., the signals produced by the brain that stimulate testosterone production).[14] It is a point of contention, but it's interesting to note.

---

12    Geoffrey L Hammond, "Plasma steroid-binding proteins: primary gatekeepers of steroid hormone action," *J Endocrinol*, 2016 Jul, 230(1): R13–R25, published online 2016 Jul 1, doi: 10.1530/JOE-16-0070.

13    Hyun-Ki Lee Joo Kyung Lee and Belong Cho, "The Role of Androgen in the Adipose Tissue of Males," *World J Mens Health*, 2013 Aug, 31(2): 136–140, published online 2013 Aug 31, doi: 10.5534/wjmh.2013.31.2.136.

14    Anand Kumar, Skand Shekhar, and Bodhana Dhole, "Thyroid and male reproduction," *Indian J Endocrinol Metab*, 2014 Jan–Feb, 18(1): 23–31, doi: 10.4103/2230-8210.126523.

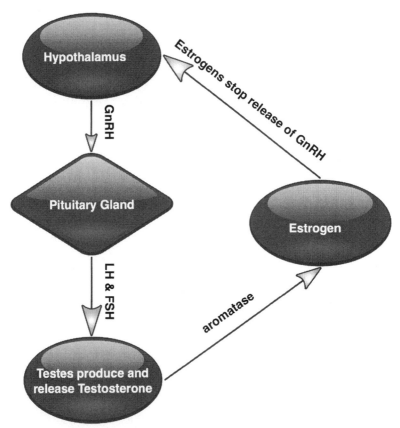

Used with permission from Balance My Hormones Ltd Copyright 2016

## THE GLOBAL EPIDEMIC OF LOW TESTOSTERONE

We are on the verge of something never seen before in the history of mankind. However, this won't be a moment to savor for our species—like the discovery of penicillin or the lunar landing. It's something much more sinister, yet virtually no one knows about it. What I refer to is the **current global epidemic of low testosterone**. The men and physicians I work with already know it's here, yet it has gone unnoticed by mainstream society.

The world has a long history of epidemics that have killed millions, from the bubonic plague to Spanish Flu. And when it's finally recognized for what it is, the epidemic of low testosterone will be up there with them. Low testosterone doesn't result in physical death, at least not immediately; instead, it consigns men to the ranks of the walking dead.

But don't take my word for it—just look around you. Our society is crumbling at the seams. Instead of living in harmony with one another and working together, we are more divided than ever. We are in a time of crisis—a crisis of masculinity. In times of crisis, men step into the breach to provide solutions. Yet most men are completely indifferent to the situation. The society they grew up in is changing beyond recognition, yet most of them prefer to watch Netflix or play Call of Duty or Fortnite. This is apathy on an unprecedented scale and is a **direct result** of low testosterone levels in society.

In 1987, Travison et al. did a seminal study to measure the testosterone levels of over 1,700 American men age 45–79. One of the unique features of this study is that it had multiple follow-ups over the course of two decades. According to the study, testosterone levels declined by 1% per year since the study began in 1987. That means a 25-year-old man in 2002 would have 15% lower testosterone than a 25-year-old man in 1987. The researchers observed a "substantial age-independent" decline in testosterone that cannot be explained by aging, health, or lifestyle factors alone, such as smoking or obesity.[15] In other words, it doesn't matter how old you are, you can be affected. The researchers hypothesized environmental factors were one of the main culprits behind this widespread decline in testosterone levels. And as we'll see later in the book, it appears they were right.

---

15    Thomas G. Travison, Andre B. Araujo, Amy B. O'Donnell, Varant Kupelian, John B. McKinlay, "A Population-Level Decline in Serum Testosterone Levels in American Men," *The Journal of Clinical Endocrinology & Metabolism*, Volume 92, Issue 1, 1 January 2007: 196–202, https://doi.org/10.1210/jc.2006-1375.

## THE MALE FERTILITY CRISIS

Between 1973 and 2011, the Hebrew University of Jerusalem undertook a landmark study on male sperm count in North America, Australia, New Zealand, and Europe. The study analyzed the sperm health of 42,935 men (a huge sample size for any scientific study), and the researchers made a startling discovery. In this 38-year period, they discovered **male sperm count declined by 50–60%!**[16] The authors of the study conclude the vast majority of men will be **infertile by 2050.** The bottom line? We could be extinct in just a few generations unless we do something about it.[17]

## WHAT IS LOW TESTOSTERONE?

Low testosterone is a condition where the body is deficient in producing testosterone. The scientific term for this is *hypogonadism*. There are two types of hypogonadism: primary and secondary. Primary hypogonadism results from a failure of the testes to produce sufficient testosterone and is typically associated with biological defects of reproductive machinery.[18,19] Although, as we'll see, the

---

16   Hagai Levine et al., "Temporal trends in sperm count: a systematic review and meta-regression analysis," *Human Reproduction Update*, Volume 23, Issue 6, 1 November 2017: 646–659, https://doi.org/10.1093/humupd/dmx022.

17   For more on male fertility, see Purusotam Basnet, Sissel A Hansen, Inger K Olaussen, Martha A Hentemann and Ganesh Acharya, "Changes in the semen quality among 5739 men seeking infertility treatment in Northern Norway over past 20 years (1993–2012)," Journal of Reproductive Biotechnology and Fertility, Volume 5: 1–7.

18   Peeyush Kumar, Nitish Kumar, Devendra Singh Thakur, and Ajay Patidar, "Male hypogonadism: Symptoms and treatment," *J Adv Pharm Technol Res*, 2010 Jul–Sep, 1(3): 297–301, doi: 10.4103/0110-5558.72420.

19   Tajar A et al., "Characteristics of secondary, primary, and compensated hypogonadism in aging men: evidence from the European Male Ageing Study," *J Clin Endocrinol Metab*, 2010 Apr, 95(4): 1810–8, doi: 10.1210/jc.2009-1796.

current epidemic of low testosterone normally stems from secondary hypogonadism (due to the environment), affecting men of all ages.

In primary hypogonadism, an individual usually has low serum (total) testosterone and high concentrations of follicle stimulating hormone (FSH) and/or luteinizing hormone (LH). The pituitary gland in the brain sees the testes not producing sufficient quantities of testosterone and responds by secreting gonadotropins (i.e., LH and FSH). However, in spite of these gonadotropins, the testes fail to respond and produce sufficient testosterone.

Secondary hypogonadism arises from an issue with the hypothalamus or pituitary gland in the brain (i.e., the areas responsible for stimulating testosterone production).[20] In secondary hypogonadism, an individual may have suffered a concussion or trauma to the head (e.g., traumatic brain injury), thereby damaging the hypothalamic pituitary axis (HPTA). This diminishes the secretion of gonadotropins (i.e., LH and FSH), resulting in low testosterone production because the signal from the brain to the testes is weak or nonexistent. In the absence of this signal, the testes fail to produce sufficient levels of testosterone. Secondary hypogonadism is characterized by low serum LH and/or FSH levels, typically below 5 mIU/L on a blood test.

So how does a physician diagnose low testosterone? In an ideal scenario, they assess the patient's symptoms along with blood tests. Typical laboratory reference ranges for serum testosterone are between 200 ng/dL and 900 ng/dL (6.9 nmol/L–34.7 nmol/L).[21] However, most physicians will make a *clinical diagnosis* of low

20   Peeyush Kumar, Nitish Kumar, Devendra Singh Thakur, Ajay Patidar, "Male hypogonadism: Symptoms and treatment," *J Adv Pharm Technol Res*, 2010 Jul–Sep, 1(3): 297–301, doi: 10.4103/0110-5558.72420.

21   Traish AM, Miner MM, Morgentaler A, Zitzmann M, "Testosterone deficiency," *Am J Med*, 2011 Jul, 124(7): 578–87, doi: 10.1016/j.amjmed.2010.12.027.

testosterone on the basis of the blood work only, regardless of symptoms. This means in order to get treatment, the patient must have testosterone levels lower than the bottom value (i.e., 6.9 nmol/L / 10.4 nmol/L). In other words, they need to be on death's door before they get treated.

## SYMPTOMS OF LOW TESTOSTERONE

The symptoms of low testosterone vary from person to person. Some men experience a few of the symptoms of low testosterone, while others experience all of them. They include:

- Anxiety
- Diminished libido
- Depression
- Lethargy
- Erectile dysfunction (ED)
- Lack of motivation and drive
- Inability to lose body fat
- Inability to gain muscle mass
- Reduced cognitive function—including hesitancy and indecisiveness

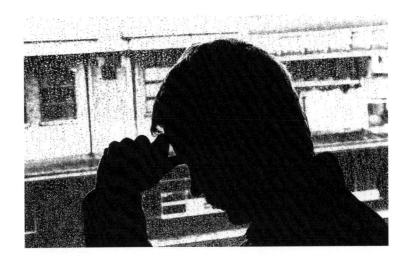

Low testosterone makes you feel like a shadow of your former self. It sucks the life out of you and deprives you of your masculinity to the point that you become a passenger in your own life.

This is not how it's meant to be; men are meant to live fulfilling lives. However, with low testosterone, this basic instinct all but evaporates. It can cause a driven, go-getting man to turn into an anxious, self-conscious wreck. Your enthusiasm for life is extinguished, and things you were once passionate about no longer move you. Now you stay at home and shut yourself off from the world.

One thing to realize is the symptoms of low testosterone do not differ by age. But the symptoms are more pronounced in young men, simply because it's like going through old age. To be clear, any diagnosis of low testosterone should go by symptoms first. However, to establish if you have low testosterone, you need to take a blood test. Now let's move on to the next chapter to find out about the type of blood tests you'll need to take.

# CHAPTER 3

## TAKING A BLOOD TEST

You think you may have symptoms of low testosterone, so it's time to get a blood test done. "But do I really need a blood test?" Yes, because without a blood test to verify your symptoms, at this stage, it's still conjecture. As the saying goes, "You can only manage what you can measure." Once you know what's going on, you're in a position to take action—whether it's changing your lifestyle or getting treatment. And if you do need medical treatment for low testosterone, your doctor will usually require at least two blood tests for validation.

You might be reading this and thinking, *I don't have the symptoms of low testosterone!* Don't wait until you have obvious symptoms of low testosterone to get a blood test. You can have the symptoms of testosterone deficiency and not even know it. This is because you can become accustomed to low testosterone without even recognizing it. Eventually, it becomes your benchmark. And you think lethargy, anxiety, and low sex drive are the norm. THEY'RE NOT!

Another thing to realize is this: People with average health don't take blood tests. You're reading this book because you want above-average health and, by extension, an above-average life. In short, you want to get optimized in every sense of the word. And part of being optimized means taking regular blood tests. Get used to the idea of taking responsibility for your own health. It's not the responsibility of your doctor, mom, spouse, or insurance company. Not only that, the more data you have on your health, the more power you have.

Unfortunately, modern healthcare is COMPLETELY reactive, and it only treats sickness when it manifests. But often by then it's too late. Instead, you need to take a proactive approach to your health. With regular blood tests, you will be able to address problems before they become an issue. And that doesn't just go for low testosterone—it means all disease.

## BLOOD TESTS: WHAT YOU NEED TO KNOW

If you're going to take a blood test, you'll also need a basic understanding of how to read it. I can hear your cries already, "But blood tests are so complex, how am I supposed to do that?" The world of blood testing can be a confusing place to the uninitiated. However, you don't need to be an expert at reading blood tests. You just need to have a sound grasp of the basics in order to make an **informed** decision about your health.

This is because most doctors know little about hormones, and even less about what constitutes optimal levels. Young men take blood tests for low testosterone and are told, "Everything is okay." But how do you know everything is okay? Just because the doctor says so? In fact, often your doctor won't even share the results with you unless you demand them.

## THE BASIC HORMONE PANEL

As a starting point to understand where your hormones are at (notice I say *hormones*, not just testosterone), you should get the following basic hormone panel done:

- Serum testosterone (total testosterone)
- Free testosterone
- Sex hormone binding globulin (SHBG)
- Luteinizing hormone (LH)
- Follicle stimulating hormone (FSH)

- Estradiol
- Prolactin
- Albumin

If you live in a country where socialized medicine is the norm (e.g., Canada or the UK), then typically you will go to your GP to get this test done. However, your GP may be unwilling to do this for you. Some doctors can be open-minded, but my experience is they are often reluctant to do extensive blood testing. This is due to cost concerns, or dismissive "I know best" attitudes leading them to tell young men they don't need a testosterone test. So your best bet is likely to get this test done at a private lab, which should be straightforward.

## WHAT THE VALUES ON A BLOOD TEST ACTUALLY MEAN

Now let's talk about this blood test and what the values actually mean. Serum testosterone, also known as total testosterone, is the total amount of testosterone in your body. However, only 2% of total testosterone is bioavailable (i.e., available for the body to use—this is known as free testosterone). Free testosterone is calculated from a mathematical formula using total testosterone, albumin, and SHBG.[22] The main factor that influences how much free testosterone your body has is your total testosterone. Essentially, the less total testosterone you have, the less free testosterone you have, although nothing in hormonal health is ever that black and white.

One common factor affecting free testosterone is the amount of SHBG in your blood. SHBG is a protein produced by the liver

---

22    Guay AT, Traish AM, Hislop-Chestnut DT, Doros G, Gawoski JM, "Are there variances of calculated free testosterone attributed to variations in albumin and sex hormone-binding globulin concentrations in men?" *Endocr Pract*, 2013 Mar–Apr, 19(2): 236–42, doi: 10.4158/EP12113.OR.

with a high affinity for sex steroids and binds strongly to testosterone.[23] Once testosterone is bound to SHBG, it's no longer available for use—hence why lab tests differentiate between free and total testosterone.

Luteinizing hormone (LH) and follicle stimulating hormone (FSH) must also be included on any hormone test to determine if primary or secondary hypogonadism is the cause of low testosterone. These hormones, also known as gonadotropins, are produced by the pituitary gland and signal the testes to produce testosterone.

Estradiol is a form of estrogen, and in men it is produced through the aromatization process via the aromatase enzyme (i.e., where testosterone is converted into estradiol). Contrary to popular belief, estrogen is not just a "female" hormone. In fact, estrogen is vital to men's health, but sadly there is still much misinformation out there. Later on in the book we'll see why estrogen is essential to male health.

Prolactin is a hormone secreted by the pituitary gland. In women, it's responsible for breast milk production, hence *pro-lactate*. The role of prolactin in men is still not fully understood, but it appears to be important in the creation of FSH and LH receptors, as well as sperm production.[24] Low prolactin levels are associated with poor sexual and psychological health.[25] Its hypersecretion (i.e., excessive

23   Hammond GL, "Access of reproductive steroids to target tissues," *Obstet Gynecol Clin North Am*, 2002 Sep, 29(3): 411–23.

24   Teresa Costa Castanhoa, Pedro Silva Moreira, Carlos Portugal-Nunes, Ashley Novais, Patrício Soares Costaa, Joana Almeida Palhaa, Nuno Sousaa, Nadine Correia Santos, "The role of sex and sex-related hormones in cognition, mood and well-being in older men and women," *Biological Psychology*, 103 (2014) 158–166.

25   Corona G et al., "Low prolactin is associated with sexual dysfunction and psychological or metabolic disturbances in middle-aged and elderly men: the European Male Aging Study (EMAS)," *J Sex Med*, 2014 Jan, 11(1): 240–53, doi: 10.1111/jsm.12327. Epub 2013 Oct 29.

production) is associated with low libido, suppressed gonadotropins, low testosterone, infertility, and erectile dysfunction.[26] It's thought to affect libido through modulating the activity of nitric oxide,[27] which is critical to blood flow to the penis and erectile strength.

Similar to SHBG, albumin is a binding and transporter protein. Although unlike SHBG, testosterone binds weakly to albumin. Its main role is to control concentrations of sex hormones in the blood; when they increase temporarily, or "when the production or function of [steroid binding proteins like] SHBG change under different physiological conditions or during disease."[28]

No one hormone takes precedence over others on a blood test because it's how they work together—not in isolation—that's important. Testing for one or two hormones doesn't tell the full story. Guys often take total testosterone-only tests and make decisions on the back of those results. But making a decision on your health with a testosterone-only test is like looking at one room in a house and buying the whole thing. You need to take a full hormone panel, **as a minimum**.

Let's say you have the symptoms of low testosterone and you take a blood test. The results show you have serum testosterone levels of 800 ng/dL (27.7 nmol/L). On paper, everything looks okay, right? However, a full hormone panel reveals you have SHBG levels of 80

26   Marinaki Maria, "The Role of Prolactin in Men," *Endocrinol Metab Syndr*, 2016, 5: 222, doi:10.4172/2161-1017.1000222.

27   Albert S. Chang, Ruriko Grant, Hirofumi Tomita, Hyung-Suk Kim, Oliver Smithies, and Masao Kakokia, "Prolactin alters blood pressure by modulating the activity of endothelial nitric oxide synthase," *Proc Natl Acad Sci U S A*, 2016 Nov 1, 113(44): 12538–12543, published online 2016 Oct 17, doi: 10.1073/pnas.1615051113.

28   Geoffrey L Hammond, "Plasma steroid-binding proteins: primary gatekeepers of steroid hormone action," *J Endocrinol*, 2016 Jul, 230(1): R13–R25, published online 2016 Jul 1, doi: 10.1530/JOE-16-0070.

nmol/L. This means despite good serum testosterone levels, most of it is bound to the SHBG. As a result, you have low free testosterone levels and the symptoms of low testosterone. The body functions as a unit, and it's the interplay of hormones that creates a picture for diagnosis—something only a full hormone panel can show. Don't skimp on blood tests.

Today, you can't afford *not* take a blood test and get your hormones checked. You no longer have the luxury of thinking low testosterone is something you will deal with when you're older. Every time you step foot outside the door, and even in your own home, you're bombarded with hazardous chemicals. From the food you eat to the water you drink to the air you breathe. There is simply no escaping it, and there is a very HIGH chance your testosterone levels have been affected. So, if you haven't already done it, make getting a test a priority.

## HOW TO READ YOUR BASIC HORMONE PANEL

As I mentioned, symptoms are the most important factor when it comes to low testosterone. Nevertheless, a thorough lab test can help provide context. The following section is a guideline for reading your basic hormone panel. But be aware this in no way, shape, or form can act as a substitution for an experienced TRT physician who can expertly interpret your results.

**Testosterone:** Research suggests low testosterone symptoms in young men can occur between with serum testosterone at 400 ng/dL (13.9 nmol/L) or below.[29] Although in practice, I have seen men with low testosterone symptoms between 500–600 ng/dL (17.3–20.8

---

29   Jason M. Scovell, Ranjith Ramasamy, Nathan Wilken, Jason R. Kovac, and Larry I. Lipshultz, "Hypogonadal symptoms in young men are associated with a serum total testosterone threshold of 400 ng/dL," Department of Urology, Baylor College of Medicine, Houston, TX, USA.

nmol/L) and sometimes more. Again this is why a testosterone test alone is useless.

**Free testosterone:** Free testosterone should consist of 2–4% of total testosterone. For example, if you have 800 ng/dL (27.7 nmol/L) of serum testosterone, you would have 16 ng/dL (2%) of free T.

**SHBG:** Ideal levels of SHBG in men are generally considered to be between 15–40 nmol/L. Low SHBG levels (i.e., below 15 nmol/L) can be caused by a number of conditions. They include hyperprolactinemia, obesity, hypothyroidism, insulin resistance, type 2 diabetes, and anabolic steroid use.[30] Low SHBG levels don't necessarily contraindicate TRT, but they must be closely monitored by your physician because it will mean you have higher levels of circulating estrogen.

Because SHBG has a high affinity for testosterone, elevated levels of SHBG, i.e. 40 nmol/L or above will reduce the amount of free testosterone in the blood. There are a number of causes of elevated SHBG levels. Estrogens and thyroxine (a thyroid hormone) are known to elevate circulating SHBG, and liver disease, obesity, insulin, and growth hormone deficiency can also increase it.[31]

Dr. John Crisler, a leading physician in hormone optimization and anti-aging, believes SHBG to be the most important assay on any lab test: "SHBG is the first thing I look at when evaluating labs, and probably spend the most time thinking about. SHBG

---

30    Megan Crawford and Laurence Kennedy, "Testosterone replacement therapy: role of pituitary and thyroid in diagnosis and treatment," *Transl Androl Urol*, 2016 Dec, 5(6): 850–858, doi: 10.21037/tau.2016.09.01.

31    Giovanni Corona, Linda Vignozzi, Alessandra Sforza, and Mario Maggi, "Risks and Benefits of Late Onset Hypogonadism Treatment: An Expert Opinion," *World J Mens Health*, 2013 Aug, 31(2): 103–125, published online 2013 Aug 31, doi: 10.5534/wjmh.2013.31.2.103.

is unquestionably the centerpiece of every proper sex hormone evaluation."[32]

**LH:** Healthy LH levels in men are considered to be 3–10 mIU/L. LH above 10 mIU/L is associated with primary hypogonadism. Levels below 5 mIU/L with resulting low testosterone is considered to be secondary hypogonadism (i.e., a failure in the pituitary gland or hypothalamus).

**FSH:** Healthy FSH ranges are generally between 3–10 mIU/L. According to research, elevated levels of FSH (above 7.5 mIU/L) are linked with low sperm count and to dysfunction in the testes (i.e., primary hypogonadism).[33] FSH levels below 3 mIU/L tend to be associated with secondary hypogonadism.

**Estradiol:** The standard estradiol reference range is 20–60 pg/mL (70-220 pmol/L). In recent times, there has been a fixation on maintaining estradiol levels within this range, and in some cases shooting for a specific number. This is because most doctors are keen to avoid unwanted side effects from high levels of estrogen. However, arbitrarily suppressing estradiol levels or "chasing numbers" can be dangerous for a number of reasons that we'll address later in this chapter. Suffice to say, recent research shows men can have estradiol levels of up to 80 pg/mL and have no symptoms of high estrogen.

Dr. Neal Rouzier suggests that it is the absence of symptoms and *not* the lab value that determines treatment for high estradiol. And according to Dr. John Crisler, traditional lab tests to measure estradiol levels in men are obsolete because they overestimate estradiol levels.

---

32   Jay Campbell, *The Testosterone Optimization Therapy Bible: The Ultimate Guide To Living A Fully Optimized Life* (Best Seller Publishing, 2018).

33   Gordetsky J, van Wijngaarden E, O'Brien J., "Redefining abnormal follicle-stimulating hormone in the male infertility population." *Ann Endocrinol (Paris),* 1999 Jul, 60(2):102-6.

So the only reliable method to test estradiol in men is via mass-spectrum liquid chromatography (i.e., a sensitive estradiol test).

This kind of test is usually only available in the United States. Therefore, patients in Canada, Europe, and other countries should be aware a standard test will tend to overestimate estradiol. This is important to understand because doctors often prescribe aromatase inhibitors (AIs) on the back of estradiol tests. In the chapter on Testosterone Replacement Therapy Protocols, we will cover AIs in more depth.

**Prolactin:** Prolactin levels below 14 ng/mL (300 mIU/L) are generally considered to be acceptable. There are several possibilities that account for elevated prolactin levels; these include SSRIs / antidepressants (e.g., citalopram) and hypothyroidism (underactive thyroid). Pituitary tumors and prolactinomas generally occur at over 47 ng/mL (1,000 mIU/L) and can sometimes produce readings of 940 ng/mL (20,000 mIU/L) or more. Elevated prolactin levels such as these must be investigated further with an MRI scan to establish if a pituitary tumor is the cause. High prolactin levels can produce symptoms of low testosterone. Therefore, prolactin must be included on any evaluation into low testosterone.

**Albumin:** The accepted range for albumin levels is 35–52 g/l. Low serum albumin levels appear to be correlated with systemic inflammation and are a predictor of disease.[34,35] However, rarely have I seen men with albumin levels that are too low or severely elevated.

34   Hiroko Ohwada, Takeo Nakayama,Yuki Kanaya, and Yuki Tanaka, "Serum albumin levels and their correlates among individuals with motor disorders at five institutions in Japan," *J Nutr Sci Vitaminol*, (Tokyo), 2007 Feb, 53(1): 37–42.

35   Klonoff-Cohen H, Barrett-Connor EL, Edelstein SL, "Albumin levels as a predictor of mortality in the healthy elderly," *J Clin Epidemiol*, 1992 Mar, 45(3): 207–12.

## FURTHER BLOOD TESTS

Taking a blood test is not just about testing for low testosterone. It's also about being proactive and monitoring your own health. Today, you can leave nothing to chance. So even if you don't have the symptoms of low testosterone, I recommend you take a blood test anyway.

Now let's imagine you take the basic hormone panel we discussed. You discover your testosterone is low, even though your other hormonal markers seem okay. If you really want to determine the cause of your low testosterone, you will require a comprehensive blood panel. In addition to any investigation into low testosterone, an in-depth test is also for completeness; to make sure your health is otherwise in good order.

Before settling on any proper diagnosis of low testosterone, it's important to get at least two tests done. And as a minimum, one of these should be a comprehensive blood panel. You need two tests because hormones can fluctuate on a day-to-day basis. And in some instances, I have seen individuals require multiple blood tests because two was not enough to establish a clear diagnosis for low testosterone. The type of blood panels and specific panels vary from lab to lab. So you may not be able to get everything I suggest here at your local lab. However, you should do your best to get as close as possible, budget permitting.

- Glucose—HbA1c, blood glucose
- Inflammatory markers—C-reactive protein, homocysteine
- Lipids—HDL, LDL, total cholesterol, triglycerides
- Liver functtkion—total protein, ALT, AST
- Kidney function—urea, eFGR, creatinine
- Thyroid function—TSH, free T3, free T4
- PSA—i.e., prostate specific antigen

- Hematology (full blood count)—hematocrit, hemoglobin, red blood cell count
- Vitamins—B12, folate, Vitamin D
- Iron markers—serum iron, ferritin, transferrin saturation, TIBC

It's not necessary for you to be able understand every one of these markers and what they mean. You just need to have an understanding of the hormonal aspect and know whether you have low testosterone or not. That's why you get a more extensive test to find out what the cause might be. In the next chapter, we will discuss what causes low testosterone.

This panel will be more expensive to obtain than a basic hormone panel; however, it's well worth it. If you have a private healthcare provider, you may even be able to get the procedure covered by insurance.

## COACHING AND CUSTOMIZED PROGRAMS

For selected 1-on-1 coaching clients who suffer the symptoms of low testosterone (e.g., lethargy, low libido, and depression), I offer comprehensive blood panels. These are offered at top-class laboratories all over the US and UK, and under the supervision of an experienced physician.

These tests go into great depth—much more than any regular test you'll get from your physician. If you do have a specific issue that's causing your hormonal imbalance (which is usually the case), we'll be able to identify it and come up with a customized nutrition, training, and supplement program to address it. In addition, we'll look to optimize lifestyle factors such as sleep. You can find out more about my 1-on-1 coaching here:

http://optimizedarmy.com/online-coaching/

## THE AVERAGE MAN AND THE "NORMAL" RANGE

Now you know what blood tests to take, it's crucial to understand the main drawback of lab tests: reference ranges. In his book *The End of Average*, author Todd Rose describes how the concept of using "normal" ranges and measuring people against predetermined averages stems from the Industrial Revolution.

During this period, to try and draw conclusions about the world, scientists began to measure things such as average birth, average weight, average complexion, and average stature. In contrast to today, at that time the average was held up as the ideal; anything that deviated from it was considered flawed. And as one scientist of the time quipped, "Everything differing from the Average Man's proportions and condition, would constitute deformity and disease."[36]

Rose goes on to cite a study done by the US Air Force to measure the average proportions and dimensions of their pilots. The idea of the study was to provide data to enable them to design a cockpit to fit these average proportions. The researchers expected a sizeable amount of 4,063 pilots in the study to fall within the "average range" in all 10 dimensions. The result? Not a single pilot had "average" proportions.[37] Therefore, if there is no average for our physical proportions, how can there possibly be one for hormone levels?

Today, you may think the idea of measuring averages is laughable, but this is how modern medicine treats patients. We're still using a 19th century solution for a 21st century problem. Most doctors treat low testosterone based on where your testosterone levels sit within the "normal" reference range. So if you're within this reference range, then as far as they're concerned, you're normal. Frankly, the idea that

---

36  Todd Rose, *The End of Average: How to Succeed in a World That Values Sameness* (HarperOne, 2016).

37  Rose, *The End of Average*.

men only merit treatment for low testosterone based on arbitrary concentrations of testosterone regardless of symptoms is a farce.

The biggest problem with these reference ranges is they're based on samples from <u>men of all ages,</u> and they're not age-adjusted. For instance, you could be a 30-year-old man with testosterone levels of 300 ng/dL (10.4 nmol/L), and that would make you "normal." But in reality, this testosterone level may be acceptable for an 80-year-old, but not for a 30-year-old in the prime of life.

***The "Normal Range" is found through purely statistical means; it has absolutely nothing to do with health and happiness. —Dr. John Crisler***

Apart from not being age-adjusted, another issue with the reference ranges is the numbers themselves keep changing. For example, let's take the reference range used by LabCorp—a well-known private blood-testing laboratory in America. As you can see from the image below, prior to July 2017, the bottom end of the range was 348 ng/dL (12.1 nmol/L).

| Previous LabCorp Reference Interval | New LabCorp Reference Interval (effective July 17, 2017) |
|---|---|
| Adult Male >18 years: 348 – 1197 ng/dL | Adult Male >18 years: 264 – 916 ng/dL |
| Comment: Adult male reference interval is based on a population of lean males up to 40 years old. | Comment: Adult male reference interval is based on a population of healthy nonobese males (BMI <30) between 19 and 39 years old. |

This means you had to have testosterone below 348 ng/dL to be considered hypogonadal (low T) and qualify for treatment. In other words, you had to be living a miserable life no man would ever want. However, as of 2017, LabCorp moved the goalposts and lowered the reference range further. So now, you must have testosterone level of 264 ng/dL (9.2 nmol/L) or lower to be classed as hypogonadal. That's almost a full 100 points lower—a HUGE difference!

Nevertheless, these changes are not restricted to the bottom end of the range. The high end of the range was previously 1197 ng/dL (40 nmol/L), an acceptable and healthy level of serum testosterone. However, as of July 2017, the top end of the range has been lowered by 281 points to 916 ng/dL (31.8 nmol/L).

This is HUGE because now testosterone levels above 916 ng/dL are considered supraphysiologic! In other words, this puts you in the same category as someone abusing steroids. So if you undergo TRT and your testosterone level rises above this threshold, your doctor may reduce your dose or threaten to withdraw treatment altogether!

This is a crazy scenario, but it's not just LapCorp doing this—it's happening in labs all over the world. LabCorp themselves take their data from a study of 9,054 men in the United States and Europe. The study concluded that a normal range for healthy, non-obese males aged 19 to 39 years is 264 to 916 ng/dL.[38] This further proves testosterone levels are plummeting.

The "normal" reference range has failed so many men. Laboratories and doctors need to come together to put forward an age-adjusted

38    Travison TG, Vesper HW, Orwoll E, Wu F, Kaufman JM, Wang Y, Lapauw B, Fiers T, Matsumoto AM, Bhasin S, "Harmonized Reference Ranges for Circulating Testosterone Levels in Men of Four Cohort Studies in the United States and Europe," *J Clin Endocrinol Metab*, 2017 Apr 1, 102(4): 1161–1173, doi: 10.1210/jc.2016-2935.

reference range. For instance, if a 25-year-old man takes a blood test, he should be able to compare it with men of his own age—NOT with an entire population of men. And not only should the reference range be age-adjusted, it should also distinguish between **average and optimal**. Because who really wants AVERAGE testosterone levels? So you can be AVERAGE like everyone else? Unfortunately, there is no solution in sight while doctors and researchers in ivory towers continue to oversee endocrinology guidelines.

## THINGS TO KNOW BEFORE TAKING A BLOOD TEST

Most physicians recommend you take a blood test first thing in the morning. This is because testosterone production peaks in the morning and drops over the course of the day. However, a "normal" testosterone test first thing in the morning can be misleading. Because if you have serum testosterone of 400 ng/dL (13.9 nmol/L) at 9 a.m., by the afternoon your testosterone levels are in the gutter. And this is exactly what happened to me.

Before testosterone replacement therapy, I had a blood test at 9 a.m. that was 345 ng/dL (12 nmol/L) and a 2 p.m. test that was 230 ng/dL (8 nmol/L). The first test was technically within the reference range, while the second test was well below. In all honesty, it doesn't really matter what time of day you take the test—low testosterone is low testosterone.

You should be careful to avoid sexual intercourse or masturbation before your blood test, because this can elevate gonadotropins, prolactin, and even PSA levels, thereby creating a false picture. You should take a blood test fasted because food can significantly affect markers such as glucose, lipids, and even testosterone.

Aim to avoid exercise up to 72 hours before taking your blood test. The stress of exercise can elevate biomarkers such as urea, creatinine, cholesterol, and hematocrit,[39] again creating a false picture of your health. I have seen men whose blood tests indicated they were on the verge of imminent kidney failure, only to find out they exercised on the day of the test. A final thing to consider is that blood tests measuring testosterone shouldn't be evaluated when you are sick, due to disruption of homeostasis.

## WHAT IS AN OPTIMAL LEVEL OF TESTOSTERONE?

For a young man, an optimal level of testosterone can be anywhere from 500–1000 ng/dL (17 nmol/L – 34.7 nmol/L). It's a wide range—but it's all about context. For instance, a 30-year-old man may feel fine at 500 ng/dL (17.3 nmol/L) of serum testosterone. Whereas a man of the same age may have the symptoms of low testosterone at 500 ng/dL (17.3 nmol/L), hence why testosterone levels alone do not tell the whole story and detailed blood tests must be done to investigate possible causes.

Men have a tendency to become fixated on numbers; whether it's how much they bench press, their testosterone level, or their macronutrient intake. Before they've even taken a test, some men tell me, "I want total testosterone of 800 ng/dL (27.7 nmol/L)." Because they read it somewhere on the Internet, they conclude that's best. So I ask them, "How do you know that number is optimal for you?" They never have a good answer because it's not the number that's important—how you FEEL is the number one guideline. That is, if you feel great and positive about life, your mood and energy are good, and you have a healthy sexual appetite, that's all there is to it. All these things are the diametric opposite of low testosterone.

Does this mean lab values are useless? Not at all—they are simply

---

39  Stacy E. Foran, MD, PhD, Kent B. Lewandrowski, MD, Alexander Kratz, MD, PhD, MPH, "Effects Of Exercise On Laboratory Test Results," *Laboratory medicine*, October 2003, number 10, volume 34.

part of a two-pronged approach, as opposed to being the *only* approach. Modern medicine lumps everyone into one group and treats them accordingly. But there is no one-size-fits-all approach when it comes to elevating testosterone; hormone optimization is still both an art and science. Nothing is black and white when it comes to human health because we are all biochemically unique. Lab values are important, but they are still **guidelines**.

As mentioned, a diagnosis of low testosterone must be validated by symptoms accompanied by a minimum of two blood tests that show you have serum testosterone of 500 ng/dL (17.3 nmol/L) or less. But what if you have serum testosterone higher than 500 ng/dL and still have symptoms? Indeed, there is a crossover of symptoms from other conditions with low testosterone, which we'll discuss in the next chapter. For example, elevated SHBG caused by hypothyroidism can lower your free testosterone, despite adequate levels of serum testosterone. Once more, this is another example of why serum testosterone tests by themselves are wholly inadequate.

## "I HAVE LOW TESTOSTERONE. NOW WHAT?"

When you have the symptoms of low testosterone and lab values to match (you did get blood work done, right?), it's time to take action. However, the first step is NOT to dive headlong into testosterone replacement therapy. This is not like taking a supplement where you experiment with it for a few weeks. Understand, using exogenous testosterone (whether prescription or anabolic steroids), you shut down your body's natural production and become reliant on it. TRT is a lifelong commitment and is not to be taken lightly.

But just because you shouldn't take it lightly doesn't mean you use it as an excuse to do nothing. Too often I've seen men find out they have low testosterone, only to do nothing. They rationalize they're "taking their time" and "thinking it over." But here's the cold reality:

**They're just scared** and likely in a state of disbelief. I understand; but pretending the problem doesn't exist won't make it go away.

Wishing it didn't happen to you at such a young age and sitting around feeling sorry for yourself won't change anything. Life is full of challenges, and you must see this as another one you have to face. In fact, you should view the diagnosis of low testosterone as positive. Because it means you know the root cause of your misery and suffering. And with this book in your hands, now you have the power to address it.

Every man who desires optimal levels of testosterone MUST lead a lifestyle that promotes it. No exceptions. In the next chapter, we'll look at things you can do to lead a testosterone-friendly lifestyle. These lifestyle changes apply both to men who want to boost their testosterone and men who are already on TRT. It doesn't matter if you take testosterone or not because a poor lifestyle will counteract the positive, life-enhancing effects of testosterone.

# INTERVIEW WITH DR. JOHN CRISLER

Dr. John Crisler is a world renowned expert on testosterone replacement therapy (TRT), having created several treatment protocols that have changed the way physicians everywhere care for their patients. There are good reasons why men have traveled from every state as well as dozens of foreign countries to be seen by him: "Dr. John" successfully treats the tough cases.

His book, *Testosterone Replacement Therapy: A Recipe for Success,* is a must-read for those who are serious about hormone optimization. Not only is it well written and informative, but it is written from the perspective of a leading physician with over 17 years of experience treating patients in the field of hormone health. Aside from testosterone optimization, Dr. Crisler also specializes in thyroid hormone optimization, adrenal fatigue, and preventive medicine. And as with the other physicians featured in this book, Dr. Crisler practices what he preaches by living a fully optimized and healthy lifestyle.

**Daniel Kelly:** Dr. Crisler, much is made of the side effects of TRT. In your opinion, are the side effects part and parcel of treatment, or can they be mitigated, if not avoided altogether?

**Dr. John Crisler:** I think if you go through a physician who knows what they're doing, the side effects are of no consequence whatsoever. There is a risk of your blood getting thicker—it's called erythrocytosis, which is a natural process for testosterone. It stimulates the bone marrow to make more red blood cells. This is not the same as polycythemia or polycythemia vera, which is a deadly disease by virtue of the fact the platelets don't work.

Platelets are what makes blood clot, and you may see blood getting thicker—the hemoglobin, and/or hematocrit may rise. We now know no one has ever died from their blood getting thick from testosterone replacement therapy. Although I hasten add that if you feel better by donating blood, it's definitely a wonderful thing to do because about 50 people get the benefits of the blood that you give. By all means, go down and do the procedure, but it's not necessary.

Some people do feel a little pressure when their blood gets too thick. So if that's the case, go ahead and donate blood. It's also good for men to dump iron out of their body by donating blood because excess iron rusts and sticks in the lining of your coronary arteries. The problem is, when you get regular blood draws, sometimes you start to get really weak and tired. Therefore, I will often check a patient's iron levels and discover they're depleted.

As part of this, I also check their ferritin levels, and ferritin is a measure of the storage of iron. If ferritin gets too low, they become weak and get shortness of breath, and conversion of thyroid hormones are inhibited. Iron does a lot more than just make red blood cells. I get into a lot of arguments with hematologists about this because they try to treat erythrocytosis or polycythemia, rather than depleting iron through blood draws, and that makes us sick because iron does a lot of stuff for our bodies as well, so you really have to look at the big picture, Daniel.

**Daniel Kelly:** There are many myths around estrogen, especially in the context of male health, and many people believe it to be a "female hormone." But how important is estrogen to men's health, and how do you monitor and manage it in your patients?

**Dr. John Crisler:** Estrogen is important for everyone's health, including men. It's crucial for maintaining bone mass, it's very important for the brain. In fact, the brain thinks so much of estrogen it makes its own! It's important for the lipid profile, cardiovascular health, and also our emotional state because the emotional component of our sexual well-being is closely associated with estrogen levels. So guys with low estrogen feel very flat with respect to their sexuality and even can cause some erectile dysfunction.

The real problem in this stage are laboratory testing issues. It's really difficult to get the proper tests because the only methodology that's valid for testing estrogen in adult males is a liquid chromatography mass spectroscopy. Most places are running the old immunoassay testing, and the immunoassay testing is often fooled by too many of what I call, "false prophets of estrogen." There are a lot of other things in the blood that look like estrogen, so these false prophets elevate the number.

The problem with that is when the doctor only treats the patient by the number on a laboratory print out, rather than actually talking to the patient. With this form of testing, the estrogen may look elevated when in reality it's not. Therefore, they may prescribe an aromatase inhibitor when estrogen wasn't high in the first place. So that trashes the estrogen in the patient, and when that happens it's very bad, it's very bad for your health, all the way round.

The question whether we should treat estrogen or not seems to be up for debate. However, the debate really stems from the fact that doctors use the wrong testing methodology. So you can't draw any conclusion to them at all. You can say nothing about the estrogen level because the testing is not valid. I mean, you're going to hang your hat on something when you don't have any valid testing.

Elevated estrogen does a lot of bad stuff for us. Estrogen is a major player in causing gynecomastia. Although growth hormone, prolactin, and progesterone can also increase it. But if guys who have sore nipples or breast tissue growth are given an AI and it goes away, that means it was the estrogen. It's as simple as that. Therefore, in my mind there's no question you need to treat it. There are no studies where an appropriate dose of an anastrozole or any other aromatase inhibitor ever hurt anybody. In fact, to my knowledge there's not a single study that's ever been done using an appropriate dose of an aromatase inhibitor. So what conclusions can we draw? None.

The people at the forefront who claim to practice evidence-based medicine really aren't. They draw **unwarranted extrapolations or conclusions** from very poorly run tests that have no basis in reality whatsoever. It's important to understand estrogen contributes not only to nipple issues and water retention, but it also increases the risk of cancer—and that has a lot to do with hormonal balance in general, as opposed to just estrogen itself.

Estrogen is actually a class of hormones, and we have identified around 40 so far. Some are good for you, some bad for you, and some of them can be modulated by using over-the-counter supplements such as calcium-d-glucarate, diindolylmethane (DIM), or its parent compound indole-3 carbinol. I use them in patients when we need to manage the balance of different estrogen hormones.

With regard to aromatase inhibitors—if you don't have symptoms of high estrogen, I don't treat it because that would be okay for that particular patient. And if his estrogen is twice the normal range, but he has no estrogen symptoms, I don't do anything about it.

In relation to estrogen, sex hormone binding globulin (SHBG) is the centerpiece of every proper hormone evaluation. If a guy has very low or lower SHBG, sometimes they can tolerate almost no estrogen. These guys have a lot of anxiety from a moderate dose of testosterone because they have so much free estrogen floating around that gives them anxiety and ramps up their sympathetic nervous system. Basically, they've got a lot of adrenaline and so forth, and they're kind of "spinning their wheels in the sand" all the time, and it burns them out.

When the patient has the symptoms of high estrogen, there's no question whatsoever in my mind that we must properly test and treat estrogen using appropriate doses. Again, if the patient doesn't have the symptoms, I don't treat. There are just too many things we don't know about yet. If it's not bothering him, I don't want to add another drug in. And sometimes, again, we can increase the metabolism or breakdown of estrogen using calcium d-glucarate, diindolylmethane (DIM), or indole-3 carbinol. This way we can clear it out and we don't really need an aromatase inhibitor, and that can work very well in some patients.

**Daniel Kelly:** Could you talk more about how you treat estrogen with calcium d-glucarate in your patients?

**Dr. John Crisler:** Broadly speaking, calcium d-glucarate keeps estrogen flowing out of the body and keeps it metabolized. It prevents the body from pushing it back into the system and prevents gut bacteria, for instance, from pushing it back into the body.

I've used 500 mg twice a day, and a lot of patients have told me their libido went through the roof when they were on a calcium d-glucarate. Although, because I had a heart attack, which was no doubt brought on by stress, it means I don't want the extra calcium in my coronary arteries, even though I take high dose vitamin K (discussed in the chapter Supplements for Young Men). The calcium d-glucarate does add around 250 mg of additional calcium a day, and I do eat enough dairy and so forth, so I don't want the extra calcium. Subsequently, I stopped taking the calcium d-glucarate, and I noticed it when I did. I have estrogen issues myself. It didn't help me a lot, but I do use indole-3 carbinol a couple of times a day.

**EDITOR'S NOTE:** Indole-3 carbinol (I3C) is closely related to diindolylmethane (DIM) and is a phytochemical derived from cruciferous vegetables, and is a negative regulator of estrogen.[40] This makes it a suitable alternative to aromatase inhibitors. And we'll discuss this topic at length in the chapter Testosterone Replacement Therapy Protocols.

There are several reasons why your estrogen can go up and cause a problem. One is that you're taking too much testosterone, so it's converting into too much estrogen, in which case the aromatase inhibitor might not be dosed right. The testosterone to estrogen conversion, which is through the aromatase enzyme, can be variable. Lots of things ramp up the aromatase enzyme, including caffeine, alcohol, and inflammatory things. Basically, everything that is bad for a man increases the conversion of testosterone to estrogen.

For instance, when I drink a lot of caffeine, I have to take a little more anastrozole (i.e., aromatase inhibitor) because I convert more testosterone to estrogen. And on a weekend when I'm out partying with the guys, I do notice my chest hurts more, my estrogen goes up, and I feel bloated and frankly, a little bitchy. In this case, I may take another 0.3 mg of anastrozole a day earlier. I take a 0.5 mg anastrozole on my two-shot days each week, so when the testosterone goes up, then the anastrozole is there to inhibit the conversion of testosterone to estrogen, and that works very well for me.

**Daniel Kelly:** Men who desperately need medical treatment may avoid testosterone replacement therapy altogether because they believe it could be harmful to their health. Although, we know low

---

40   Auborn KJ, Fan S, Rosen EM, Goodwin L, Chandraskaren A, Williams DE, Chen D, Carter TH, "Indole-3-carbinol is a negative regulator of estrogen," *The Journal of Nutrition*, 2003 Jul;133(7 Suppl):2470S-2475S.

testosterone is actually more harmful to your health. Could you talk a little bit about this?

**Dr. John Crisler:** Testosterone is really only good for a man; individually, and as a society, no question about it. Currently, there's a big scare about increased cardiovascular disease risk with testosterone, but we know that's completely bogus. Ultimately, it's being driven by a bunch of greedy lawyers and doctors who have no idea what they're doing.

However, my friend Dr. Abraham Morgentaler looked at one of the major studies on it and simply took out his calculator, added up the numbers on it, and discovered they didn't even have the numbers right! And the so-called "world-class" peer-reviewed medical journal that posted that garbage study refused to print a retraction. So there is an agenda there against testosterone, mostly by foolish politicians who link it to steroid use and so on—but these are two different things. Comparing testosterone replacement therapy to doing steroids is like drinking a glass of wine compared with a fifth of liquor: "The dose makes the poison," as they say.

Other potential side effects of testosterone include blood thickening, and we've clarified that isn't really a problem. Gynecomastia is another, but again that's equally manageable. Several different things can cause gynecomastia. If someone has it, in addition to looking at prolactin, you've got to stop their growth hormone and peptides because they can contribute to it.

**EDITOR'S NOTE:** Elevated prolactin levels are often associated with gynecomastia and can suppress gonadotropins such as luteinizing hormone. It's thought elevated estrogen levels can elevate prolactin levels, although it's not clear whether prolactin itself is responsible for breast tissue growth in men.

Prostate health is another cause for concern. With regards to this, we now use something called the *saturation model*, and I invite readers to look that up. What this means is, if your testosterone is over 200 ng/dL (6.9 nmol/L), any amount of testosterone is going to help you because it's important to saturate the receptors. They have even developed protocols for patients to actually take high doses of testosterone when they have prostate cancer. Although it really depends on what your testosterone is when you start.

In future, I think we'll see more therapeutic applications for high levels of testosterone. However, not many doctors know how to manage high-dose testosterone, so it will be a question of educating them.

We have been completely wrong about this all these years about testosterone and its applications. Old ideas are hard to break, so you have to keep an open mind about everything and be willing to throw things out when they prove to be untrue. And oftentimes our own egos get in the way of progress.

**Daniel Kelly:** Given that testosterone therapy is so new and cutting-edge, how does someone discern fact from fiction, and what's a good or bad study from a physician's point of view?

**Dr. John Crisler:** Doctors tend to practice medicine by mere titles of studies. If you read the abstract, most of us rarely go through the study. I'm not qualified to make a statistical analysis of a center study—mathematicians do that—but applying good old-fashioned farmer's logic takes you a long way. You have to ask yourself, "Are we really testing something that is practical?"

For example, several years ago they did a study using Testim (a 2% testosterone gel). And they started out giving twice the usual starting dose to men who already had high blood pressure. They didn't even monitor estrogen, much less treat it. So, of course, blood pressure went up in many subjects. As a result, they stopped the study and put a black box warning on testosterone. But that's absolute foolishness. Where do you ever see twice a starting dose of any medication used in studies? So there's bias there, and there was no monitoring. This is what happens when people who have no idea what they're doing conduct scientific studies.

If they're honest enough to admit it, for many in academia it's about seeking grant money and producing in order to keep their job. It's not about producing results that have any resemblance to reality, and there are studies regarding endocrinology (i.e., the study of hormones) that are garbage. The statistical analysis of numbers really does not work in epidemiology (i.e., the study of disease).

In the foreword to my book, the one and only Dr. Eugene Shippen says you can't apply classical epidemiology to endocrinology because everyone is biochemically unique. It's almost like we are trying to compress all of humanity into a monolithic creature. The fact of the matter is, we are all different. You know, everyone has their own sweet spot for testosterone, for estrogen, for every hormone. And finding that sweet spot is what the master physician does. It can be different for everybody. Like in our previous example of the guy who has high estrogen—that might be okay for him. If he has no symptoms, then it's likely fine for him.

You have to talk to your patients to see how they're doing. Epidemiology is going to fail because the so-called testosterone "normal range" **has absolutely nothing to do with health and happiness**. Elsewhere in medicine, if you're in the "normal range" you're pretty much okay, but this does not apply to testosterone.

There was a study some years ago from Cambridge University where they followed 10,000 men for 10 years. They found that of all the guys in the normal [testosterone] range, the guys in the lowest quarter of normal compared to highest quarter of normal, were 41% more likely to have died from all causes. That would sound alarm bells in any other area of medicine, but not here because there is a bias against testosterone! So why do those men with low normal testosterone die early? The joke is now, "Because they wanted to!"

**Low testosterone is not okay, and low normal testosterone is not okay.** There are guys who do great at 450 ng/dL (15.6 nmol/L), and if that works for you then that's great. But consider the normal range is 95% of the population, along with the bottom 2.5% and top 2.5%. So if a normal range goes to 1,000 ng/dL (34.7 nmol/L), that means there are guys above that too.

Sometimes guys get confused because they do a blood test and their testosterone is 500 ng/dL (17.3 nmol/L). That means they're mid-range on the test, right? No, what it really means is that's half the testosterone their body was <u>meant to run on</u>. Then the problem becomes finding a physician who understands these things.

Such a high percentage of the population has low testosterone, yet it's classed as normal. The analogy I give when I'm lecturing is that it would be like taking a potassium level out of a kidney failure patient on the way into dialysis. In patients with kidney disease, the potassium is very high, so they undergo kidney dialysis to get rid of the potassium. Yet they would never collect that potassium level and throw that in the pool to use for the "normal range" number. So why are we doing that with low testosterone?

Endocrinology is uniquely stupid in that we don't apply common sense applications used elsewhere in medicine. For instance, the half-life of a drug is never considered. We still have doctors giving these massive shots every two or three weeks, and they don't care about the half-life. So, the guy is on a really high steroid dose the first week, but the second week he's actually below baseline. It's a cruel thing to do to put your patients on this emotional and physical roller-coaster.

There are even patients out there who can only handle 50 mg a week. They're going to clinics and getting 200 mg a week and it's blowing them out. For them, that dose is four times too high. Less drugs is always better and less expensive, and that's a win-win for everybody.

**Daniel Kelly:** The difference between being at the lower and top end of the "normal" range is night and day. However, there seems to be a propensity in modern medicine for people to be average or normal. If you're average or as long as you're "within range" then that's okay. But if you want to live a high quality life, average isn't going to cut it. Could you talk about this mindset that medicine has toward being average?

**Dr. John Crisler:** Who wants to have a low normal career, a low normal income, then go on a low normal vacation? Men are meant to win. Men are meant to dominate and to succeed. They're meant to take care of their families and to do the right thing. When your testosterone is low, you just don't have much gas in your tank.

Life is hard enough as it is, and having low testosterone is like tying both your hands behind your back. The optimized life is definitely the life to live.

**Daniel Kelly:** TRT is still very much in its infancy; subsequently, patients must be selective in their choice of physician. In your opinion, what should patients look for when choosing a physician?

**Dr. John Crisler:** You've got to find out how they practice. Talk to people they've treated. Do they have a good reputation? Online reviews are ridiculous because people put up dumb stuff on the message boards. Here are some questions to ask yourself:

- Are they using hCG and using low dose hCG appropriately?
- Are they using aromatase inhibitors?
- Are they monitoring estrogen properly?
- Are they into optimizing, as opposed to just getting you into the normal range?

If they're willing to prescribe testosterone replacement therapy in the first place, that's a step in the right direction. But you really want an expert, somebody who is experienced. Although, you can be experienced and have been in practice only a few years, so it depends on context.

# CREATING A LIFESTYLE CONDUCIVE TO HEALTH

After reading this chapter, you should understand how important it is to take regular blood tests to "get under the hood" of your health. I want you to adopt a proactive mindset and preventive approach when it comes to your health. Unfortunately, most people in society are completely reactive when it comes to their health.

They remain in blissful ignorance about their own health. To my mind this is utter madness—nothing could be more important. But most behave as if health was *optional.* When these people are struck down by illness, they think they are cursed or that it's an act of God.

So in their eleventh hour, these people look to doctors as their savior. However, they could have avoided the situation in the first place by taking preemptive care of their health. In order to avoid being among their number, it's necessary that you create a lifestyle conducive to health. And at the heart of your health is optimal testosterone levels. Join me in the next chapter to learn about how to live a testosterone-friendly lifestyle.

# CHAPTER 4

# HOW TO LIVE A TESTOSTERONE-FRIENDLY LIFESTYLE

The sad truth today is that the lifestyles of most young men are horrendous. They stay up all night playing video games and watching the latest "MUST WATCH" series. As a result, they are chronically sleep deprived, overweight, depressed, and overall in a bad state of health. And when it comes to testosterone levels, living this kind of life is like driving a car on fumes when the gas tank is empty—it won't get far.

Not only this, the amount of crap the average guy eats on a daily basis is unbelievable. Breakfast is a bowl of cereal; at lunchtime it's McDonalds or a burrito with salsa and all the trimmings if they're feeling adventurous; dinner is a microwavable meal. This is the kind of food that makes their grandmothers have heart attacks. Junk food is like a one-two punch combo: it's calorically dense and devoid of micronutrients. The result is increased body fat and a dramatic and negative effect on hormone synthesis.

Next is the fact most young guys drink alcohol like it's going out of style. The typical week for most guys goes like this; Grind away and work hard all week to make money and support themselves, then when the weekend rolls around, guess what—it's PARTY TIME! That means time drinking themselves to oblivion! To be fair, they're not totally at fault for this behavior due to subliminal programing from a society enamored with alcohol. Alcohol destroys your health, and in a moment, we'll see why it's toxic to testosterone levels.

Poor lifestyle habits are the number one reason testosterone levels are at an all-time low. In your quest to boost testosterone or enhance the effects of testosterone replacement therapy, you should always look to improve your lifestyle. Stop looking to quick fixes, supplements, and drugs. Get your own house in order first. You cannot live a life of optimal health without a lifestyle to support it. Fixing your lifestyle is one of the quickest and simplest—not to mention cheapest— ways to boost your testosterone. I have seen men more than double testosterone levels after making a concerted effort to improve their lifestyle. It's more than possible, but it takes work.

In this chapter, we'll look at strategies you can use in order to lead a testosterone-friendly lifestyle. Understand that everything here is interlinked. What this means is that when you address one thing, it has a domino effect on everything else. For example, two of the strategies I advocate are prioritizing sleep and reducing stress. So when you sleep more, you reduce stress, and so on. Keep these synergies in mind while you read this chapter.

## ELIMINATE CIGARETTES, DRUGS, AND ALCOHOL

Smoking cigarettes, taking drugs, and drinking alcohol might work if you're a rock star. But you will NEVER succeed in being fit and healthy, let alone raising your testosterone, if you live this way. I sometimes wonder if the party lifestyle I lived for years contributed to low testosterone in my late 20s. In any case, I figured I could counteract the negative effects of partying by going to the gym regularly and eating a good diet. But guess what? It didn't work. You cannot live an extreme lifestyle and hope to cancel it out by going extreme in the other direction. These substances are way too powerful to be negated by diet and exercise alone, so they must be eliminated. Most men don't need me to tell them how bad cigarettes and drugs are for their health, but they're much more reluctant to give up alcohol.

For many men, alcohol is a crutch to hide the insecurity they feel about themselves, in social situations, or both—although they would never like to admit this. Instead, they rationalize excessive drinking: "Alcohol is fun!" "You gotta enjoy life!" I wonder, though, are these their opinions, or are they parroting slick marketing campaigns from beverage companies? And it's amazing to see how defensive people become when you tell them you don't drink. Society glorifies alcohol so that it's apparently impossible to have fun in a social setting without it.

When it comes to living a testosterone-friendly and fit lifestyle, alcohol is kryptonite. It results in male feminization (i.e., enlarged breasts and excess body fat, due to the phytoestrogen content). It's also a testicular toxin, lowering sperm count and causing fertility abnormalities.[41]

One study measured the effect of alcohol on testosterone levels and oxidative stress (where free radicals can damage cells and DNA), comparing 46 male alcoholics aged 20-40 years with a control group of 55 males the same age. The researchers found significantly lower serum testosterone and gonadotropin (i.e., LH, FSH) levels in the alcoholic group when compared with the control group.

They also found high levels of oxidative stress and systemic inflammation in the alcoholic group. Serum (total) testosterone levels were negatively correlated (i.e., lower) with the duration of alcohol abuse. This appears to be due to the oxidative damage on the Leydig and Sertoli cells (responsible for sperm production) in the testes and impaired function of the hypothalamic pituitary axis (HPTA).[42]

---

41   Judith S. Gavaler, Ph.D., "Alcoholic Beverages as a Source of Estrogens," *Alcohol Health & Research World,* 228 Vol. 22, No. 3, 1998.

42   M. Maneesh, Sanjiba Dutta, Amit Chakrabarti and D.M. Vasudevan, "Alcohol abuse-duration dependent decrease in plasma testosterone and antioxidants in males," *Indian J Physiol Pharmacol,* 2006; 50 (3): 291–296.

Many reading this may think their alcohol intake wouldn't be classed as "alcoholic" because they don't drink every day. However, waiting until Friday and Saturday and proceeding to drink like a fish is just as bad.

Research suggests moderate alcohol consumption has protective cardiovascular effects.[43] However, in my experience, people are quick to jump on any evidence that alcohol can be beneficial to validate their decision to drink. Testosterone improves mental clarity, whereas alcohol dulls the senses. Personally, I have a few drinks in the year for one-off celebrations, but 99% of the time I don't touch it. As far as I'm concerned, alcohol adds nothing to my life. If you give up alcohol, you may worry people think you're weird for not drinking. But guess what? People respect you when you choose not to drink **because deep down, they wish they could do the same**.

HOW TO DO IT: Stop hanging out with losers whose sole purpose is to take drugs or get drunk. You owe them no loyalty if they bring you down, and you are the average of the people you hang around with. There are plenty of successful people out there who prefer to look after their mind and body to going YOLO at the weekend. Find other activities that don't involve going to dive bars. If you have to drink to entertain clients, try to minimize your intake. However, aim to change it in the long run—no job is worth your health.

## LOSE BODY FAT AND CLEAN UP YOUR DIET

One of the major causes of low testosterone is obesity. Indeed, it's no secret that most people in our society are either overweight or obese. In America alone, it's predicted 51% of the population will be

---

43   Raj Lakshman, Mamatha Garige, Maokai Gong, Leslie Leckey, Ravi Varatharajalu, and Samir Zakhari, "Is alcohol beneficial or harmful for cardioprotection?" *Genes Nutr*, 2010 Jun, 5(2): 111–120, published online 2009 Dec 13, doi: 10.1007/s12263-009-0161-2.

obese by 2030.[44] So what's the link between obesity and testosterone? Obesity results in high estrogen levels (estrogen dominance), which can cause symptoms of low testosterone and lower sperm levels. This is because the aromatase enzyme—responsible for the conversion of testosterone to estradiol—is abundant in adipose (fat) tissue. Therefore, at higher levels of body fat, more testosterone gets converted into estrogen.

High levels of circulating estrogen can inhibit the secretion of luteinizing hormone (LH) and follicle stimulating hormone (FSH), which stops the testes from receiving the signal to produce testosterone. It can also result in the degeneration of testicular tissue, preventing proper testosterone production.[45] Obesity results in insulin resistance, and several studies show a positive correlation between insulin resistance (i.e., where cells don't respond properly to insulin) and low testosterone.[46] The mechanism by which insulin resistance lowers testosterone is not fully understood. Although it's thought to derive from excess adipose tissue and the subsequent leptin release.

Adipose tissue performs metabolic and endocrine functions in the body through the secretion of hormones and peptides, one of which is leptin. Leptin is produced in adipose tissue and is stimulated

---

44   Finkelstein EA, Khavjou OA, Thompson H, Trogdon JG, Pan L, Sherry B, Dietz W, "Obesity and severe obesity forecasts through 2030," *Am J Prev Med*, 2012 Jun, 42(6): 563–70, doi: 10.1016/j.amepre.2011.10.026.

45   Myles Leavy, Matthias Trottmann, Bernhard Liedl, Sven Reese, Christian Stief, Benjamin Freitag, John Baugh, Giulio Spagnoli, and Sabine Kölle, "Effects of Elevated β-Estradiol Levels on the Functional Morphology of the Testis - New Insights," *Sci Rep*, 2017, 7: 39931, published online 2017 Jan 3, doi: 10.1038/srep39931.

46   Nelly Pitteloud, MD, Vamsi K. Mootha, MD, Andrew A. Dwyer, BA, Megan Hardin, BA, Hang Lee, PHD, Karl-Fredrik Eriksson, MD, Devjit Tripathy, MD, DM, Maria Yialamas, MD, Leif Groop, MD, PHD, Dariush Elahi, PHD and Frances J. Hayes, MB, BCH, BAO, "Relationship Between Testosterone Levels, Insulin Sensitivity, and Mitochondrial Function in Men," *Diabetes Care*, 2005 Jul, 28(7): 1636–1642, https://doi.org/10.2337/diacare.28.7.1636.

through insulin release. Among other things, it helps regulate reproductive function, energy expenditure, and appetite suppression.[47] Leptin acts at all levels of testosterone production, and the Leydig cells in the testes themselves have multiple leptin receptors.[48] Several studies show a correlation between leptin levels and testosterone,[49] and studies of male rats show testosterone production is inhibited by high concentrations of leptin. These concentrations are similar to the levels seen in obese men.[50] Being overweight results in insulin and leptin resistance, leading to low testosterone and infertility in men.[51] So from the resultant leptin and excess estrogen alone, obesity is like a double whammy for your testosterone.

One reason obesity is rampant in our society is due to terrible diet. Most people eat a typical "Western diet" (i.e., high in saturated fat, red meat, and sugar; low in fruit, vegetables, seafood, and poultry). And that's not to mention all the preservatives and emulsifiers in the foods. This type of diet destroys the delicate balance of gut flora (i.e., friendly gut bacteria) in your intestines. It's amazing to think that gut flora plays an integral role in metabolism, immunity, behavior,

47    Havel PJ., "Role of adipose tissue in body-weight regulation: mechanisms regulating leptin production and energy balance," *Proc Nutr Soc*, 2000 Aug, 59(3): 359–71.

48    Hyun-Ki Lee, Joo Kyung Lee, and Belong Cho, "The Role of Androgen in the Adipose Tissue of Males," *World J Mens Health*, 2013 Aug, 31(2): 136–140, published online 2013 Aug 31, doi: 10.5534/wjmh.2013.31.2.136.

49    Behre HM, Simoni M, Nieschlag E, "Strong association between serum levels of leptin and testosterone in men," *Clin Endocrinol* (Oxf), 1997 Aug, 47(2): 237–40.

50    Nelly Pitteloud, Megan Hardin, Andrew A. Dwyer, Elena Valassi, Maria Yialamas, Dariush Elahi, Frances J. Hayes, "Increasing Insulin Resistance Is Associated with a Decrease in Leydig Cell Testosterone Secretion in Men," *The Journal of Clinical Endocrinology & Metabolism*, Volume 90, Issue 5, 1 May 2005: 2636–2641, https://doi.org/10.1210/jc.2004-2190.

51    David Landry, Frank Cloutier, Luc J. Martin, "Implications of leptin in neuroendocrine regulation of male reproduction," Reproductive Biology, Volume 13, Issue 1, March 2013: 1–14, https://doi.org/10.1016/j.repbio.2012.12.001.

and function of the gastrointestinal tract. Research on mice even suggests these bacteria play a role in hormone secretion and testosterone production.[52] Therefore, the importance of looking after your gut health in the context of hormones cannot be overemphasized.

In addition to looking after gut health, you should also understand the role specific foods play in testosterone production. Cholesterol has been demonized in recent years, yet it's a necessary precursor for testosterone, and adequate fat intake is necessary for testosterone production. Both human and animal studies show a positive correlation between dietary fat intake and testosterone levels.[53,54] One study looked at the effect of extra virgin olive oil and virgin argan oil (made from a tree found in Morocco) on androgen levels (i.e., male sex hormones) of 60 male volunteers age 23–40 years old. After three weeks of taking argan and olive oil, each group experienced a 19.9%

52    Hadar Neuman, Justine W. Debelius, Rob Knight, Omry Koren, "Microbial endocrinology: the interplay between the microbiota and the endocrine system," *FEMS Microbiology Reviews*, Volume 39, Issue 4, 1 July 2015: 509–521, https://doi.org/10.1093/femsre/fuu010.

53    Volek JS, Kraemer WJ, Bush JA, Incledon T, Boetes M, "Testosterone and cortisol in relationship to dietary nutrients and resistance exercise," *J Appl Physiol* (1985), 1997 Jan, 82(1): 49–54.

54    Hurtado de Catalfo GE, de Alaniz MJ, Marra CA, "Influence of commercial dietary oils on lipid composition and testosterone production in interstitial cells isolated from rat testis," *Lipids*, 2009 Apr, 44(4): 345–57, doi: 10.1007/s11745-008-3277-z.

increase and 18.5% increase in total testosterone levels respectively.[55] [56]

Whatever diet you choose, you should be careful to avoid refined carbohydrates that lead to spikes in blood sugar. One study looked at the effect of 75g oral glucose administration on glucose levels and sex hormones. Blood samples were taken at 0, 30, 60, 90, and 120 minutes after ingestion. The authors of the study found glucose ingestion significantly reduced total and free testosterone, regardless of how subjects processed glucose itself.[57]

You should also aim to restrict your intake of dietary gluten where possible. People who experience an immune reaction to gluten (i.e., from wheat, barley, rye) tend to have celiac disease. However, research suggests there is also a condition known as non-celiac gluten sensitivity (NCGS) that shares many of the symptoms of celiac disease. These include brain fog, nausea, bloating, and fatigue. These symptoms sound similar to low testosterone, right? Well, research suggests gluten can elevate prolactin levels,[58] which can

55   Derouiche A, Jafri A, Driouch I, El Khasmi M, Adlouni A, Benajiba N, Bamou Y, Saile R, Benouhoud M, "Effect of argan and olive oil consumption on the hormonal profile of androgens among healthy adult Moroccan men," *Nat Prod Commun*, 2013 Jan, 8(1): 51–3.

56   For more on the negative effects of a Western diet, especially in regard to carbohydrates, see Jeremy Silva, "The effects of very high fat, very low carbohydrate diets on safety, blood lipid profile, and anabolic hormone status," *J Int Soc Sports Nutr*, 2014, 11(Suppl 1): 39, published online 2014 Dec 1, doi: 10.1186/1550-2783-11-S1-P39.

57   Caronia LM, Dwyer AA, Hayden D, Amati F, Pitteloud N, Hayes FJ, "Abrupt decrease in serum testosterone levels after an oral glucose load in men: implications for screening for hypogonadism ," *Clin Endocrinol* (Oxf), 2013 Feb, 78(2): 291–6, doi: 10.1111/j.1365-2265.2012.04486.x.

58   Delvecchio M, Faienza MF, Lonero A, Rutigliano V, Francavilla R, Cavallo L, "Prolactin may be increased in newly diagnosed celiac children and adolescents and decreases after 6 months of gluten-free diet," *Horm Res Paediatr*, 2014, 81(5): 309–13, doi: 10.1159/000357064.

cause many of the symptoms of low testosterone and interfere with libido in particular.

<u>HOW TO DO IT</u>: Improve gut health by eliminating processed foods and sugar from your diet. I usually refrain from making blanket statements on macronutrient ratios because every person is unique and has different health goals. However, most would do well to have a moderate amount of carbohydrates to fuel performance, enough protein for building muscle and repairing tissue, and sufficient fat for health and testosterone synthesis.

Low-carb diets are suitable for the vast majority of the population, simply because our sedentary lifestyles do not require a high amount of carbohydrates. Prior to the Industrial Revolution, we required more calories (including carbohydrates), to fuel physically demanding jobs. But today this is no longer the case. Furthermore, most people simply cannot process carbohydrates that well, so they end up feeling sluggish. At the time of writing, I myself have been following a ketogenic diet. The results have been incredible. This type of diet may be too extreme for many, but I encourage you to look into it.

Aim to increase dietary fat intake primarily through monounsaturated and polyunsaturated fats. Foods rich in these types of fats include nuts, seeds, avocados, and fish (avoid vegetable oils like the plague!). With regard to carbohydrates, aim to eat low glycemic, complex sources, such as lentils, brown rice, sweet potatoes, and oatmeal. Protein is fundamental to living a fit lifestyle, so make sure you eat enough. Excellent sources of protein include fresh fish (e.g., salmon), ground beef, chicken, turkey, and whole eggs.

**Fat distribution is genetically determined and hormonally regulated. —Russ Scala**

## LIFT WEIGHTS

Lifting weights must form a core part of your life. Although some guys say, "But I prefer cardio!" Good luck staying weak then! Honestly, since when did it become fashionable to be a pussy? You don't have to become the World's Strongest Man, but to be clear, as a man, you're MEANT TO BE STRONG. And if you want to be strong, you've got to lift weights. Get this idea out of your head that lifting is only for "meatheads."

Most young men don't exercise, let alone lift weights. If you're a man and not exercising on a regular basis, you're doing yourself a huge disservice. Aside from the health benefit, the incredible advantage you will have over your peer group by lifting weights **cannot be understated**. It will give you energy and confidence in yourself to make big moves while your competition falls by the wayside. It will also help you develop discipline and build your character. All for the price of a monthly gym membership—that's an exponential ROI.

Lifting weights will help you lose body fat and gain muscle. Studies show serum testosterone can rise immediately after resistance training,[59] although the literature is conflicting on whether resistance training elevates resting testosterone levels. One study looked at the effects of an eight-week heavy resistance-training program in untrained men and women. Hormone samples were taken pre- and post-training, and at follow-up points over the study. After six

59   Hooper DR, Kraemer WJ, Focht BC, Volek JS, DuPont WH, Caldwell LK, Maresh CM. "Endocrinological Roles for Testosterone in Resistance Exercise Responses and Adaptations," *Sports Med,* 2017 Sep, 47(9): 1709–1720, doi: 10.1007/s40279-017-0698-y.

weeks, the men showed an increase in total testosterone.[60] However, it remains unclear whether the effect on hormone profiles would be the same in trained individuals.

And what about the type of training routine? It appears training protocols high in volume, with moderate to high intensity and short rest periods, are best for raising testosterone levels (bodybuilding style) versus low-volume, high-intensity protocols with long rest intervals (powerlifting style).[61]

HOW TO DO IT: There are many free training programs on the Internet and thousands of YouTube videos you can watch—so you have no excuse whatsoever. Go to the gym today and **do something**. Imperfect action is better than no action. Read the chapter Building Your Body with Testosterone for an overview.

And if you don't have any idea where to start, find a gym buddy (preferably one who is stronger than you), or hire a coach like me to help you. The Internet is a great resource for educating yourself. However, many guys mistakenly consider themselves experts after reading a few ebooks and watching videos on training. I see guys who spend months or years training but make little to no progress. Yet they shirk the idea of investing in a coach. If you want to speed up your success, then working with a coach is one of the best things you can do. It means you gain access to their knowledge and experience, which might take you years to obtain by yourself. Personally, I have invested thousands of dollars to work with coaches in all areas of my life, and it's always proved to be an invaluable investment.

---

60   Kraemer WJ, Staron RS, Hagerman FC, Hikida RS, Fry AC, Gordon SE, Nindl BC, Gothshalk LA, Volek JS, Marx JO, Newton RU, Häkkinen K, "The effects of short-term resistance training on endocrine function in men and women," *Eur J Appl Physiol Occup Physiol*, 1998 Jun, 78(1): 69–76.

61   Kraemer WJ1, Ratamess NA, "Hormonal responses and adaptations to resistance exercise and training," *Sports Med*, 2005, 35(4): 339–61.

## REDUCE STRESS

In modern life, stress can come in many forms; pressure at work, psychological stress, and physical stress. These stressors are often exacerbated by our addiction to electronic devices. Today, we are constantly connected to the world through smartphones; chronically jacked up so that our brains don't get the chance to switch off. Numerous studies have demonstrated the negative effects of smartphones on health and stress levels.[62]

One study looked at the effects of smartphone use on psychological behavior and cognition (i.e., judgment, decision-making, etc.). Over the course of three months, it compared users with minimal smartphone use to those with heavy smartphone use. They found heavy smartphone use was associated with increased impulsivity, reduced cognition, and hyperactivity.[63] Another study looking at smartphone use among 688 university students concluded that frequent smartphone use was positively associated with symptoms of depression, anxiety, daytime fatigue, and decreased sleep quality.[64] And as we'll see shortly, sleep deprivation is bad news for your testosterone.

Chronic stress can affect metabolic pathways and the immune system. It can also increase biological aging; the net result is increased

---

62   Michitaka Yoshimura, Momoko Kitazawa, Yasuhiro Maeda, Masaru Mimura, Kazuo Tsubota, and Taishiro Kishimoto, "Smartphone viewing distance and sleep: an experimental study utilizing motion capture technology," *Nat Sci Sleep*, 2017, 9: 59–65, published online 2017 Mar 8, doi: 10.2147/NSS.S123319.

63   Aviad Hadar, Itay Hadas, Avi Lazarovits, Uri Alyagon, Daniel Eliraz, Abraham Zangen, "Answering the missed call: Initial exploration of cognitive and electrophysiological changes associated with smartphone use and abuse," *PLoS ONE*, 12(7): e0180094, https://doi.org/10.1371/journal.pone.0180094.

64   Jocelyne Matar Boumosleh, Doris Jaalouk, "Depression, anxiety, and smartphone addiction in university students—A cross sectional study," *PLoS One*, 2017, 12(8): e0182239, published online 2017 Aug 4, doi: 10.1371/journal. pone.0182239.

oxidation. Indeed, it appears oxidative damage over time to the Leydig cells in the testes plays a key role in low testosterone.[65] This oxidative damage is typically associated with aging males. However, this aging process is accelerated today due to the poor lifestyles of many young men. Therefore, oxidative damage to the testes from stress is quite plausible and may explain the incidence of low testosterone among many young men.

Cortisol is a well-known stress hormone and is associated with stress. Elevated cortisol levels can result in poor cognitive performance and lead to memory loss. It also appears high estradiol levels (e.g., resulting from high body fat) can interact with cortisol to heighten feelings of stress. Chronic stress is also strongly associated with obesity and metabolic disease.[66,67]

HOW TO DO IT: Stress is part of life, but that doesn't mean you have to let it ruin your health and lower your testosterone. Disconnect from technology regularly and aim for a lifestyle that minimizes stress. Do things that calm your mind. What works for some people, doesn't always work for others. Experiment with different things and find out what works for you. Perhaps going for walks in the forest is your thing. Maybe you find meditating, swimming, or watching a movie is relaxing for you. Get rid of toxic people and energy vampires in your life—that's something every man can benefit from.

---

65   M.C. Beattie, L. Adekola, V. Papadopoulos, H. Chen, and B.R. Zirkin, "Leydig Cell Aging and Hypogonadism," Exp Gerontol, 2015 Aug, 68: 87–91, published online 2015 Feb 18, doi: 10.1016/j.exger.2015.02.014.

66   Helen Lavretsky and Paul A. Newhouse, "Stress, Inflammation and Aging," Am J Geriatr Psychiatry, 2012 Sep, 20(9): 729–733, doi: 10.1097/JGP.0b013e31826573cf.

67   Mousumi Bose, Blanca Oliván, and Blandine Laferrère, "Stress and obesity: the role of the hypothalamic–pituitary–adrenal axis in metabolic disease," Curr Opin Endocrinol Diabetes Obes, 2009 Oct, 16(5): 340–346, doi: 10.1097/ MED.0b013e32832fa137.

## PRIORITIZE SLEEP

There are no two ways about it; the quality of your sleep informs the quality of your waking life. So a good night's rest should be high up on your list of priorities. In today's world, though, sleep is among the lowest priorities. There is a price to pay when you don't sleep enough. Insufficient sleep increases inflammatory markers, leading to accelerated aging and disease. Inflammation is the underpinning of disease.

Lack of sleep activates certain gene pathways that contribute to conditions such as diabetes, heart disease, and atherosclerosis. It is also associated with obesity, insulin resistance, and elevated blood pressure. Difficulty falling asleep is also associated with higher risk of cardiovascular death.[68,69]

Sleep deprivation can lower hormonal markers including thyroid, testosterone, and growth hormone. One study looked at the effect of one week of sleep deprivation on the testosterone levels of 10 healthy men. The average age of the group was 24.3 years old, and each participant slept for five hours each at night. Indeed, this is actually a typical night's sleep for 15% of the US working population! The researchers found testosterone levels were decreased 10–15% after the sleep deprivation period.[70] This study was not that strong, given

68   Michael R. Irwin et al., "Sleep Loss Activates Cellular Inflammatory Signaling," *Biol Psychiatry*, 2008 Sep 15, 64(6): 538–540, published online 2008 Jun 17, doi: 10.1016/j.biopsych.2008.05.004.

69   Janet M. Mullington, Ph.D., Norah S. Simpson, Ph.D., Hans K. Meier-Ewert, M.D., and Monika Haack, Ph.D., "Sleep Loss and Inflammation," *Best Pract Res Clin Endocrinol Metab*, 2010 Oct, 24(5): 775–784, doi: 10.1016/j.beem.2010.08.014.

70   Rachel Leproult, PhD and Eve Van Cauter, PhD, "Effect of 1 Week of Sleep Restriction on Testosterone Levels in Young Healthy Men," *JAMA*, 2011 Jun 1, 305(21): 2173–2174,

doi: 10.1001/jama.2011.710.

it was only a week long—but it gives you an idea. Now, imagine the effect of chronic sleep deprivation on your testosterone!

It comes as no surprise to anyone with poor sleep habits that sleep deprivation can lead to decreased cognition, diminished working and long-term memory, and impaired visual performance. It can also lead to more rigid thinking and poor decision-making.[71] Later on in the book, we'll see how vital testosterone is to cognitive performance.

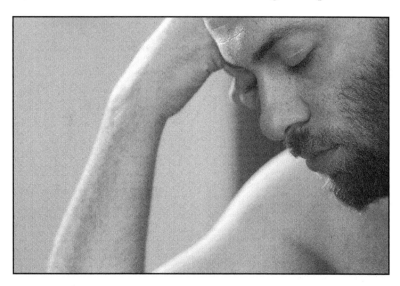

Research also suggests obesity is strongly associated with sleep loss. Lack of sleep promotes high concentrations of ghrelin—a peptide secreted from the stomach that stimulates appetite. Long periods without sleep result in increased appetite, particularly for foods high in carbohydrates, and excessive caloric intake. Furthermore, the elevation of evening cortisol levels due to chronic sleep loss is likely to lead to the development of insulin resistance.[72]

---

71   Paula Alhola and Päivi Polo-Kantola, "Sleep deprivation: Impact on cognitive performance," *Neuropsychiatr Dis Treat*, 2007 Oct, 3(5): 553–567.

72   Eve Van Cauter, PhD; Kristen Knutson, PhD; Rachel Leproult, PhD; Karine Spiegel, PhD, "The Impact of Sleep Deprivation on Hormones and Metabolism," *THE LANCET*, Vol 354, October 23, 1999.

The good news is the negative impact of sleep deprivation, particularly on your endocrine system, can be reversed relatively quickly by getting plenty of rest. One interesting study looked at the metabolic and hormonal effects of "catch-up" sleep in men with chronic, lifestyle-driven sleep deprivation. The study involved 19 men with an average age of 28.6 years with at least six months' history of lifestyle-driven sleep restriction. The subjects spent three days in a laboratory, which mimicked the catch-up sleep these men regularly did on weekends. The researchers found that three days of catch-up sleep increased insulin sensitivity and testosterone, compared to sleep deprivation.[73] Nevertheless, I want to stress that living your life by the seat of your pants Monday to Friday, then making up for it at the weekend is NOT conducive to long-term health.

HOW TO DO IT: The foundation of good sleep is proper sleep hygiene. This means creating an environment conducive to restful sleep. You should aim to change your bedsheets regularly, ensure your room is pitch black, and maintain a cool temperature when you go to sleep. Also make sure you have a comfortable mattress. I spent several months in Asia, where they believe hard mattresses are good for your back. Being used to Western comforts, I found this was really rough on my back. After that experience, I've grown to appreciate the importance of a comfortable mattress.

Another factor is exposure to blue light emitted from electronic devices. It's best to avoid blue light exposure before bed. Ideally, you should stop using any devices 60–90 minutes before bedtime. There is now compelling evidence that blue light LED exposure could

---

73    Killick R, Hoyos CM, Melehan KL, Dungan GC 2nd, Poh J, Liu PY, "Metabolic and hormonal effects of 'catch-up' sleep in men with chronic, repetitive, lifestyle-driven sleep restriction," *Clin Endocrinol* (Oxf), 2015 Oct, 83(4): 498–507, doi: 10.1111/cen.12747.

affect glucose metabolism.[74] Better sleep will result in improved testosterone levels, and improved testosterone levels will result in better sleep.

## HOW LONG SHOULD YOU SPEND IMPROVING YOUR LIFESTYLE AND RAISING YOUR TESTOSTERONE?

The primary cause of low testosterone is a poor lifestyle. Therefore, the more time and effort you invest into improving your lifestyle, the better your chances of raising your testosterone. Many men I encounter feel terrible with low testosterone, so they look to TRT as their savior in the same way a religious fanatic seeks salvation. Yet they do nothing about the lifestyle that led to low testosterone in the first place. Understand, if you haven't created the right lifestyle, **it does not matter** if you take testosterone.

Take a few moments to answer the questions below. You must be able to answer yes to the majority of them to know if you're on track with your lifestyle. If you can't do that, you have <u>no business</u> undergoing testosterone replacement therapy or looking at a medication to solve your problems. **Clean up your lifestyle first.**

- Do you sleep between 7–8 hours a night?
- Do you eat a nutritious diet consisting mainly of whole foods?
- Have you minimized or eliminated alcohol?
- Do you exercise regularly and lift weights?
- Do you have body fat of 15% or lower?
- Do you get enough sun exposure?

Most men think their diet is "pretty good." However, when I ask them to track everything that goes into their mouth, they see with

---

74   Ivy N. Cheung, Phyllis C. Zee, Dov Shalman, Roneil G. Malkani, Joseph Kang, and Kathryn J. Reid, "Morning and Evening Blue-Enriched Light Exposure Alters Metabolic Function in Normal Weight Adults," *PLoS One*, 2016, 11(5): e0155601, published online 2016 May 18, doi: 10.1371/journal.pone.0155601.

stark clarity how bad it actually is. Guys come to me all the time asking about testosterone replacement therapy. But after a few questions, I discover they haven't even tracked their food intake. You must track what you eat for a period of 2-3 months to see how your body responds. I recommend using a free food tracking app like My Fitness Pal.

When it comes to improving their lifestyle and raising testosterone, men typically have two questions. The first is: *How long does it take to see the results of lifestyle improvements?* In truth, there are no black-and-white answers because everyone has a different starting point. It depends on how low the testosterone is to begin with and how bad the lifestyle is that caused it.

Some guys require major lifestyle overhauls, whereas others may need to make a few tweaks. There is no way to accurately predict or guarantee how a change in lifestyle will affect testosterone levels. I've seen every possible scenario. I've seen men who've done a complete 180 on their lifestyle and seen a dramatic increase in their testosterone. I've worked with men who live a clean lifestyle, yet still fail to raise their testosterone. Nevertheless, after making changes to their lifestyle, most men tend to see improvements.

The second question men have is: *How long should I spend improving my lifestyle before looking for treatment?* You should spend a minimum of three months on this. And even then, that's not usually long enough. Depending on the severity of the case, it may take up to six months or more to get your testosterone into the optimal range. This gives you enough time to adjust to your new habits and observe any improvement in symptoms. Beyond that, it's likely your issue is medical rather than lifestyle-related. Make sure you take a blood test prior to embarking on any lifestyle changes to monitor the effects.

Take another blood test three months later to compare your testosterone levels before and after you made changes.

Your ability to increase your testosterone through lifestyle change will be determined by what caused the low testosterone in the first place. If the root cause is from chronic stress, being overweight, and eating garbage, then low testosterone is typically reversible. On the other hand, if your endocrine system is compromised after abusing anabolic steroids for years, lifestyle changes will likely be ineffective. We will cover this topic in depth in the chapter Young Men and the Anabolic Steroid Epidemic.

The success of your lifestyle changes is reduced further given the amount of testosterone-lowering chemicals in our environment. According to Dr. Rob Kominiarek, fewer than 20 out of 100 men ages 30–50 will be able to reach upper quartile (optimal) hormone levels through lifestyle changes alone. He also says it "takes a truly disciplined type-A individual to implement this type of recovery plan."[75] But that's not to say it's impossible.

To maintain any hope of optimizing your endogenous (natural) testosterone levels, you must be 100% committed to living a testosterone-friendly lifestyle. That means you need to go all out. Unlike the stuff you read on the Internet, you can't hack your way to great health. It takes discipline and sacrifice to lead this kind of lifestyle, yet the rewards are immense. I won't lie to you, though, this lifestyle is not for everyone.

If lifestyle changes fail to relieve symptoms *and* elevate blood testosterone levels, you need to get more specific and find out what else may be causing your low testosterone. This is why I recommend getting a detailed blood panel up front versus only getting a hormone

---

75   Campbell, *The Testosterone Optimization Bible.*

panel. Even though it's more expensive, it will save you time and money in the long run.

Context is everything when increasing your testosterone levels. For example, you may be able to boost your total testosterone from 300 to 400 ng/dL (10.4–13.9 nmol/L) through lifestyle changes alone. However, it's unlikely this kind of increase will result in relief of symptoms. And in this scenario, there are a couple of things at play. Either you have a medical issue, which requires testosterone replacement therapy, or there is another condition that is causing your low testosterone. In the next chapter, we'll look at the potential causes of low testosterone.

# INTERVIEW WITH PAUL BURGESS

Now you should have a good overview of what it means to lead a testosterone-friendly lifestyle. In my experience, most guys can get the exercise part down. However, many struggle with the diet aspect of their lifestyle. It can be confusing and overwhelming at times trying to decipher all the information on the Internet about dieting. As a result, the subject is largely misunderstood.

To this end, I chose to interview Paul Burgess. I consider him an expert in nutrition and many of the other topics discussed in this chapter. Paul is the owner of Athletic Fitness & Nutrition and has been coaching clients in training and dieting for over 20 years. He is a Clinical Nutritionist and has diplomas in Anti-Aging and Advanced Personal Training.

**Daniel Kelly:** Paul, one of the biggest trends in the health and fitness industry nowadays is ketogenic dieting. What is your view on the ketogenic diet and who should do it?

**Paul Burgess:** The ketogenic diet is hugely misunderstood. It was originally designed to treat drug-resistant epilepsy in children, but 99% of people using it now do not have this problem. Therefore, the extremes of a ketogenic diet tend not to work that well for them.

In my opinion, the majority of people have normal genetics for carbohydrate metabolism. That means they can handle carbohydrates well at a normal level. Here is where perspective is VERY important.

NORMAL levels of carbohydrates are around 75–100 g a day for most people. But since the advent of the high-carb, low-fat diet in the 1950s, our perspective has been skewed to believe normal levels are more like 300–400 g a day. Some people can handle high carbohydrate intake as they have the genetics to deal with them, but the majority of us are not able to do so effectively.

So, when designing a nutrition plan for someone, it is important to assess their individual carbohydrate tolerance and adjust accordingly. For some, a very low carbohydrate intake of under 30 g a day may work (as in the ketogenic diet), but you tend to lose a lot of essential nutrients when doing this. As a result, a slightly higher level of around 75–100 g tends to work well for most people to keep their blood glucose under control and weight in check while giving them good energy levels, better sleep, improved cognitive function, and overall well-being.

**Daniel Kelly:** I understand you look into blood tests, organic acid tests, and food intolerance tests with your clients. Why do you consider these tests important? And how will taking these tests impact the diet you set for a client versus an off-the-shelf plan?

**Paul Burgess:** Testing a client's blood is an amazing tool to know exactly what is going on at a cellular level. If we have that information, then we can be much more specific when designing the most appropriate nutrition plan. We can still produce very good bespoke plans without it, but it takes a bit of trial and error to get it right, whereas using testing cuts straight to the chase and also shows us any particular health issues that may need support from the nutrition side of things, which we may not see without the testing.

**Daniel Kelly:** Given you think we should reduce our carbohydrates intake, what type do you recommend?

**Paul Burgess:** As I mentioned earlier, carbohydrates work well in the right amounts. Choosing low-glycemic sources of carbs like oats, sweet potatoes, and root vegetables all work well. There is a fair amount of carbohydrate in non-starchy vegetables, so if you eat the right amount of vegetables on a daily basis, there is often no need to go heavy on starchy carbs.

However, if we are looking at performance and recovery, it would be different. Training hard is not a normal daily activity (even though many people do it), and may require more carbohydrates to facilitate performance and recovery. Again, this would need to be assessed on an individual basis. Remember, though, consistent hard training is not good for long-term health optimization.

**Daniel Kelly:** What should people eat in terms of pre- and post-workout nutrition? And what is your opinion on pre-workout boosters and post-workout shakes?

**Paul Burgess:** Depending on the activity, you will probably only need your normal nutrition to fuel most workouts. I would say 90% of people who go to the gym and train **do not train anywhere near** the intensity needed for specialized pre- and post-workout nutrition. If you are one of the 10% that do, then using a few extra carbs beforehand would be beneficial. Post-workout, I would not have anything for about an hour then eat a meal with some omega-6 fats in it to increase the inflammation you have created in the workout.

I advise this because the higher the inflammation you can create, the more adaption you will get from the workout. Just be sure to have a high omega-3 anti-inflammatory meal later in the day or the following day. There is no need for protein shakes, especially whey protein. They cause gut issues in most people, as well as spiking blood sugar, causing insulin to spike and the body to potentially store fat. Stick with eating protein from food sources.

Pre-workout formulas can have a benefit when you train. They help open up the blood vessels and get more nutrients to the cells while training. This is obviously dependent on you having a nutrient-dense diet in the first place. A non-caffeinated version would be my preference, as some are **overloaded with caffeine for no reason**.

**Daniel Kelly:** Are there any specific supplements you would recommend young men to take? And given that the supplement industry is unregulated, how can you know what you're getting is good quality or not?

**Paul Burgess:** Without testing someone to see if they are deficient in anything, the basic supplements I would recommend are:

- Vitamin D
- A good multivitamin
- L-Carnitine

And, most importantly, X-Cell nucleotides. Visit https://shop.mfit.com/products/x-cell_to see why these are so useful. Quality is definitely something to be concerned about. Ultimately, you get what you pay for, so you could use a practitioner to order pharmaceutical-grade products to be sure. This method will be quite expensive, though.

# CHAPTER 5

# FURTHER CAUSES OF LOW TESTOSTERONE

Guys say to me all the time, "I didn't know it was important to know about testosterone!" In an ideal world, we would never need to go hunting for a diagnosis. We'd leave it to the professionals, so to speak. **But we live in a world that is far from ideal for human health,** and this won't change anytime soon. So you can choose to bury your head in the sand, or you can do something about it.

Let's imagine you have the symptoms of low testosterone, and you've taken a blood test to validate them. At the end of the previous chapter, I said you need to rule out any underlying causes that can be addressed before seeking medical treatment (i.e., TRT). This chapter is going to serve as your low testosterone "checklist." That is, if you've already improved your lifestyle with recommendations from the previous chapter, yet you fail to see improvement in your symptoms, you must rule out others causes.

If you address these causes and cut the head off the snake, hopefully you won't have to undergo testosterone replacement therapy for the rest of your life. However, there are no guarantees—everyone's circumstances are unique. Don't get me wrong, I am a massive advocate of TRT because it can create such positive change in your life. **But it should only be used by those who need it;** you should aim to avoid a lifelong treatment whenever possible.

## VITAMIN AND MINERAL IMBALANCES

Vitamins and minerals are micronutrients responsible for countless biological functions including metabolism, bone production, cognition, and hormone synthesis. Vitamins are organic substances, the majority of which cannot be made by the body, and are mostly obtained through food. They are classified into two categories: fat-soluble and water-soluble. Examples of fat-soluble vitamins include vitamins D and K, with the only water-soluble vitamins being vitamins B and C. Minerals are inorganic substances. Minerals are also classified into two categories: macrominerals and trace minerals (microminerals). Examples of macrominerals include magnesium and electrolytes, such as calcium and sodium. Trace mineral include iron, selenium, and zinc.

When it comes to health and fitness, most people focus on their macronutrient intake (i.e., fats, carbohydrate, and protein). "It's all about the macros, bro!" However, micronutrients are critical to your health, and failing to get sufficient quantities of them, due to a poor diet or medical condition, can lead to disease—especially low testosterone. This is why it's vital to get adequate intake through your diet and ensure you make up any shortfall with supplementation. Correct supplementation has become even more critical in recent years, given the fact that many foods (organic or otherwise) lack sufficient micronutrients. Nonetheless, you cannot hope to raise your testosterone through supplementation if your diet is poor. Concentrate on eating a good diet before you look at supplements. Below are examples where a micronutrient imbalance may affect testosterone levels. Although it's important that you understand it's often a combination of factors that lead to low testosterone, it's unlikely one *single* micronutrient is to blame.

Guys ask me every day about the best supplements to boost

testosterone. But the fact is, the human body doesn't work like that. And so if you supplement with one of the following micronutrients, that doesn't necessarily translate into boosting your testosterone. However, you do have a great chance if you correct micronutrient deficiencies in conjunction with the lifestyle changes discussed in the previous chapter.

- **Vitamin D.** Studies show association between vitamin D levels and serum testosterone levels. One study looked at the effect of vitamin D supplementation on testosterone levels. Participants (54 men in total) received either 3,332 IU of vitamin D or a placebo daily for one year. All participants had a deficiency in vitamin D and low testosterone levels, as confirmed by blood tests. Researchers noted a significant increase in baseline serum testosterone and free testosterone in the vitamin D group compared to the placebo group.[76]

- **Zinc.** There is strong evidence to suggest zinc deficiency can also lead to low testosterone. One rodent study looked at the effect of a zinc-deficient diet compared with a control group on hormone concentrations. Rats with zinc deficiency showed lower concentrations of gonadotropins and serum testosterone. They also showed increased aromatization [conversion] of testosterone to estradiol,[77] resulting in higher estrogen levels. This demonstrates yet another mechanism by which men can develop low testosterone and become estrogen dominant.

---

76    Pilz S, Frisch S, Koertke H, Kuhn J, Dreier J, Obermayer-Pietsch B, Wehr E, Zittermann A., "Effect of vitamin D supplementation on testosterone levels in men," *Horm Metab Res*, 2011 Mar, 43(3): 223–5, doi: 10.1055/s-0030-1269854.

77    Om AS, Chung KW, "Dietary zinc deficiency alters 5 alpha-reduction and aromatization of testosterone and androgen and estrogen receptors in rat liver," *J Nutr*, 1996 Apr, 126(4): 842–8.

It's important to note that zinc only appears to improve hormonal profiles <u>when there is a deficiency</u>. So in the absence of any deficiency, it's unlikely to do much. Zinc is a common ingredient in many testosterone booster formulations, such as ZMA. One particular study looked at the effect of ZMA supplementation on training adaptations and anabolic hormones in young, resistance-trained men. The researchers noted no significant differences in body composition or hormones in the control group versus the supplementation group.[78]

- **Selenium.** Selenium is a naturally occurring mineral found in water and some foods. It helps make proteins called antioxidant enzymes that protect against cell damage. It also plays an important role in metabolism and thyroid function. Low levels of selenium are associated with increased prevalence of thyroid disease.[79] And we'll see in a moment how proper thyroid function is integral to testosterone production.

Nevertheless, it appears selenium's role is not limited to thyroid regulation alone. Selenium is important to testosterone metabolism, and research suggests selenium can actually enhance testosterone production in the Leydig cells. Optimizing your selenium levels (and the other things listed

78   Colin D Wilborn, Chad M Kerksick, Bill I Campbell, Lem W Taylor, Brandon M Marcello, Christopher J Rasmussen, Mike C Greenwood, Anthony Almada, and Richard B Kreider, "Effects of Zinc Magnesium Aspartate (ZMA) Supplementation on Training Adaptations and Markers of Anabolism and Catabolism," *J Int Soc Sports Nutr*, 2004, 1(2): 12–20, published online 2004 Dec 31, doi: 10.1186/1550-2783-1-2-12.

79   Qian Wu, Margaret P. Rayman, Hongjun Lv, Lutz Schomburg, Bo Cui, Chuqi Gao, Pu Chen, Guihua Zhuang, Zhenan Zhang, Xiaogang Peng, Hua Li, Yang Zhao, Xiaohong He, Gaoyuan Zeng, Fei Qin, Peng Hou, Bingyin Shi, "Low Population Selenium Status Is Associated With Increased Prevalence of Thyroid Disease," *The Journal of Clinical Endocrinology & Metabolism*, Volume 100, Issue 11, 1 November 2015: 4037–4047, https://doi.org/10.1210/jc.2015-2222.

here) by itself is unlikely to change your testosterone levels. My aim is to show you how different pieces of the jigsaw fit together. Correcting micronutrient deficiencies is just part of your strategy—not the whole strategy.

## FUNGAL INFECTIONS AND PARASITES

There is anecdotal evidence and research to suggest fungal infections can impact the endocrine system at multiple levels, ultimately leading to hypogonadism (low testosterone). Fungal infection can directly damage testicular tissue and lower fertility.[80] A common type of fungal infection that can affect men and women in equal measure is yeast infection. Fungus and yeast are present in every person. It is part of our microbiome and is needed to maintain proper digestive and restorative function. It is only when you have an overgrowth of the microorganisms—or a particular strain that is pathogenic—that the problems occur. You will often see fungal/yeast infections present themselves as athlete's foot, jock itch, a persistent clearing of the throat, brain fog, bloating, and much more. Treatment can come in the form of natural herbs and enzymes like oregano oil and saccharomyces boulardii, or antifungal medications like fluconazole.

Research suggests that, in addition to fungal infections, parasites such as roundworm and tapeworm can cause endocrine disorders. Multiple animal studies have shown parasitic infection to affect sex hormone production (i.e., lower testosterone) and dramatically affect sexual behavior. Anecdotally, in humans it can cause fatigue, joint pain, and anxiety.

Treatment for parasites such as tapeworm typically involve an oral

---

80    Michail S. Lionakis, MD, ScD, George Samonis, MD, Dimitrios P. Kontoyiannis, MD, MS, ScD, "Endocrine and Metabolic Manifestations of Invasive Fungal Infections and Systemic Antifungal Treatment," *Mayo Clin Proc*, 2008 Sep, 83(9): 1046–60, doi: 10.4065/83.9.1046.

medication, such as Biltricide, which paralyzes it. Androgens also play a protective role in the immune system and can combat parasite infection. Experimental treatment in rodents with androgens, such as DHEA, DHT, and testosterone, lead to decreased parasite infection. In contrast, treatment with estradiol (E2) increased infection threefold, and insulin appeared to stimulate parasite production.[81,82] Indeed, it appears estradiol is crucial for parasite growth. In male mice, infection with tapeworm increased estradiol concentrations to 200 times normal, while decreasing testosterone levels by 90%, resulting in feminization of the mice.[83] This has profound implications because it means many men may unknowingly be perpetuating parasitic infection through their lifestyle. That is, estrogen dominance from poor lifestyle choices and frequent insulin spikes from processed, carbohydrate-rich foods.

If you've already done a battery of tests to look into the symptoms of your low testosterone, particularly fatigue; yet there is no clear cause, then it may be worth evaluating for parasite and fungal infection.

---

81   Romel Hernández-Bello, Ricardo Ramirez-Nieto, Saé Muñiz-Hernández, Karen Nava-Castro, Lenin Pavón, Ana Gabriela Sánchez-Acosta, and Jorge Morales-Montor, "Sex Steroids Effects on the Molting Process of the Helminth Human Parasite Trichinella spiralis," *Journal of Biomedicine and Biotechnology*, Volume 2011, Article ID 625380, 10 pages, http://dx.doi.org/10.1155/2011/625380.

82   Karen Nava-Castro, Romel Hernández-Bello, Saé Muñiz-Hernández, Lorena López-Griego, Jhonatan A. Hernández-Valdés, Valeria López-Salazar, Nelly Tiempos-Guzmán and Jorge Morales-Montor, "Neuroimmunoendocrine Interactions in Murine Cysticercosis: From the Lab Bench Work to Its Possible Applications in Controlling Porcine Cysticercosis and Human Neurocysticercosis, Novel Aspects on Cysticercosis and Neurocysticercosis Humberto Foyaca Sibat," *IntechOpen*, January 30, 2013, DOI: 10.5772/50700, http://www.intechopen.com/books/novel-aspects-on-cysticercosis-and-neurocysticercosis/neuroimmunoendocrine-interactions-in-murine-cysticercosis-from-the-lab-bench-work-to-its-possible-ap.

83   Larralde C, Morales J, Terrazas I, Govezensky T, Romano MC, "Sex Hormone Changes Induced by the Parasite Lead to Feminization of the Male Host in Murine Taenia crassiceps Cysticercosis," *J Steroid Biochem Mol Biol*, 1995 Jun, 52(6): 575–80.

This can be done through a urine organic acid test (OAT). Organic acids are metabolic byproducts of cellular metabolism that are excreted through urine. These tests can help identify problems with infection, metabolism, and inflammation. Abnormally high levels of organic acids may indicate infection. Organic acid tests can be useful for when traditional blood tests show everything is "normal," yet you still don't feel right.

## THYROID DYSFUNCTION

The thyroid gland is a hormone gland located in the front of the neck, below the voice box. It plays a key role in metabolism and growth. It also regulates crucial biological functions such as energy expenditure, thermogenesis, and muscle contraction.[84,85]

Thyroid disorders are becoming increasingly common, and this is in no small part due to the prevalence of endocrine disruptors in our environment—discussed in the next chapter. The most common endocrine disease is primarily hypothyroidism (i.e., thyroid deficiency due to abnormality in the thyroid gland. This is characterized by high levels of thyroid stimulating hormone (TSH), and low concentrations of thyroxine (T4).[86] Whereas hyperthyroidism (i.e., overactivity of the thyroid gland) is characterized by high levels of TSH and low levels of thyroxine (T4) triiodothyronine (T3).[87]

84    Bloise FF, Cordeiro A, Ortiga-Carvalho TM, "Role of thyroid hormone in skeletal muscle physiology," *J Endocrinol*, 2018 Jan, 236(1): R57–R68, doi: 10.1530/JOE-16-0611.

85    Domenico Salvatore, Warner S. Simonides, Monica Dentice, Ann Marie Zavacki, and P. Reed Larsen, "Thyroid hormones and skeletal muscle—new insights and potential implications," *Nat Rev Endocrinol*, 2014 Apr, 10(4): 206–214, published online 2013 Dec 10, doi: 10.1038/nrendo.2013.238.

86    Ali J Chakera, Simon HS Pearce, and Bijay Vaidya, "Treatment for primary hypothyroidism: current approaches and future possibilities," *Drug Des Devel Ther*, 2012, 6: 1–11, published online 2011 Dec 22, doi: 10.2147/DDDT.S12894.

87    Birte Nygaard, "Hyperthyroidism (primary)," *BMJ Clin Evid*, 2008: 0611, published online 2008 Mar 25.

So what do thyroid issues have to do with testosterone? Animal studies show thyroid hormones can stimulate testosterone production, and both hypo and hyperthyroidism can affect testosterone production in men. Hypothyroidism is associated with low SHBG levels and low total testosterone. It can lead to elevated prolactin levels, which can also produce the symptoms of low testosterone. In comparison, hyperthyroidism can increase SHBG, total testosterone (due to elevated SHBG, so the body compensates), and it can also increase the aromatization (i.e., conversion) of testosterone to estrogen, resulting in estrogenic symptoms such as moodiness and gynecomastia and can ultimately lead to sexual dysfunction.[88,89]

Many of the symptoms of thyroid dysfunction mimic those of low testosterone, including depression, inability to lose weight, anxiety, and low libido. But despite being a common endocrine disorder, thyroid dysfunction is often overlooked and misdiagnosed. Subsequently, it's possible to misdiagnose someone with low testosterone when, in fact, the real culprit is thyroid dysfunction.

To rule out the possibility of thyroid dysfunction in your low testosterone, you should take a thyroid function test. Most doctors rely solely on thyroid stimulating hormone (TSH) as a marker of thyroid health; however, evidence suggests TSH by itself is inadequate. Your thyroid function test should include the following:

- TSH
- Free T3
- Free T4

---

88  Megan Crawford and Laurence Kennedy, "Testosterone replacement therapy: role of pituitary and thyroid in diagnosis and treatment," *Transl Androl Urol*, 2016 Dec, 5(6): 850–858, doi: 10.21037/tau.2016.09.01.

89  Anand Kumar, Skand Shekhar, and Bodhana Dhole, "Thyroid and male reproduction," *Indian J Endocrinol Metab*, 2014 Jan–Feb, 18(1): 23–31, doi: 10.4103/2230-8210.126523.

If your thyroid function has impacted your testosterone levels, you would address it the same way as you would low testosterone (i.e., through improving diet and lifestyle factors). And depending on severity, it may involve thyroid medication. Once again, as with testosterone medication, you want to avoid taking thyroid medication where possible.

## IRON OVERLOAD AND HEMOCHROMATOSIS

Iron is a trace mineral essential to multiple biological processes, including oxygen transport, cognitive function, immune system function, and the formation of red blood cells. Iron requires its own section due to the prevalence of iron-related conditions and the effect it can have on hormone levels. Iron concentration in the body is highly regulated, and in excessive amounts it can form free radicals, leading to tissue damage. Research shows iron overload can damage cells in the testes, ultimately leading to hypogonadism.

Hemochromatosis is an iron overload disorder that is characterized by high elevated transferrin saturation (>45%) and serum ferritin levels (>300 ug/L). The condition is classified into two categories: primary and secondary hemochromatosis. Primary hemochromatosis is genetic, accounting for up to 90% of cases.[90] Secondary hemochromatosis can result from conditions such as anemia, alcoholic liver disease, and chronic liver disease like hepatitis C. Iron overload can impact the endocrine system and testosterone production. It appears nearly half of men affected with hemochromatosis suffer from low testosterone symptoms, including erectile dysfunction and low libido.[91]

90  Bacon BR, Adams PC, Kowdley KV, Powell LW, Tavill AS, "Diagnosis and management of hemochromatosis: 2011 practice guideline by the American Association for the Study of Liver Diseases," *Hepatology*, 2011, 54(1): 328–343.

91  Nazanin Abbaspour, Richard Hurrell, and Roya Kelishadi, "Review on iron and its importance for human health," *J Res Med Sci*, 2014 Feb, 19(2): 164–174.

for iron overload is through a blood test that includes uration, ferritin, serum iron, and total iron-binding BC). If these markers are elevated, further testing ranted, including a genetic test for hereditary hemo-chroma... .s. In the case of iron overload from hemochromatosis, typical treatment involves iron depletion therapy [i.e., therapeutic phlebotomy (blood draw)]. The research on iron depletion therapy and its effect on low testosterone is sparse. However, it appears thera-peutic phlebotomy can help restore sexual function and sex hormone concentrations in some men with hereditary hemochromatosis.[92]

## FURTHER CAUSES OF LOW TESTOSTERONE

There are further potential causes of low testosterone (both primary and secondary hypogonadism).

- **Undescended testicles.** Also known as cryptorchidism. Prior to birth, the testicles develop in the abdomen and then move down to their place in the scrotum. However, in certain cases, one or both testes may fail to descend at birth. This condition affects approximately 3% of full-term and 30% male infants. However, in 80% of cases, the testes descend by the third month of life.[93]

  Treatment for this condition may involve a short-term dose of hCG (discussed later in the book), or luteinizing hor-mone-releasing hormone. If left untreated, it can result in hypogonadism and lack of masculinizing features, such as facial hair growth and a low voice.

---

92    Thomas M Kelly, M.D., Corwin Q Edwards, M.D., A. Wayne Meikle, M.D., James P Kushner, M.D., "Hypogonadism in Hemochromatosis: Reversal with Iron Depletion," *Annals of Internal Medicine*, 101(5): 629–32, December 1984.

93    Stephen W. Leslie, Carlos A. Villanueva, "Cryptorchidism," *Treasure Island* (FL): StatPearls Publishing; 2018 Jan.

- **Klinefelter syndrome.** This condition results from an abnormality of the X and Y sex chromosomes. Normally, males have one X and Y chromosome. However, with Klinefelter's, males may have two or more X chromosomes. This additional X chromosome can lead to underdevelopment of the testes, resulting in low libido, erectile dysfunction, and infertility.

  Klinefelter's is one of the most common chromosome disorders, with an incidence of 0.1% to 0.2% in newborn male infants. Testosterone treatment is typically given to patients with this condition while they are young to ensure proper masculine development.[94,95] This condition is often overlooked and misdiagnosed by doctors and patients alike due to lack of knowledge; consequently, some individuals are not diagnosed until later in life.

- **Trauma to the testes.** An injury to one or both testicles may lead to hypogonadism. This may occur due to an impact (e.g., from sports) or from conditions such as testicular cancer.

- **Traumatic Brain Injury (TBI).** This is an injury to the brain caused by a trauma to the head. This may be from an accident or fall, and the condition is commonly seen in war veterans after suffering injury in combat. TBIs can lower a number of hormonal markers, including testosterone, IGF-1, growth hormone, and luteinizing hormone. And because these hormones are neuroprotective, this can negatively impact

---

94   Nieschlag E, "Klinefelter syndrome: the commonest form of hypogonadism, but often overlooked or untreated," *Dtsch Arztebl Int*, 2013 May, 110(20): 347–53, doi: 10.3238/arztebl.2013.0347.

95   Christian Høst, Anne Skakkebæk, Kristian A Groth, Anders Bojesen, "The role of hypogonadism in Klinefelter Syndrome," *Asian J Androl*, 2014 Mar–Apr, 16(2): 185–191, published online 2014 Jan 20, doi: 10.4103/1008-682X.122201.

rehabilitation.[96] Typical treatment for a TBI can involve physiotherapy, speech therapy, neuropsychological, and cognitive behavioral therapy—often involving multiple medications.

The significance of hormones to TBI rehabilitation is often discounted. This is for a number of reasons—mainly due to ignorance on the application of hormone therapy. But it is mostly because modern medicine is compartmentalized. The cardiologist looks at the heart, and the neurologist looks at the nervous system. Therefore, they rarely take into account the entire equation.

This is madness when you consider the human body works as an entire unit. To find out more about this topic, I recommend you read Andrew Marr's excellent *Tales From the Blast Factory*, written from the perspective of a veteran on how debilitating a TBI can be, and how optimal testosterone levels can restore health.

- **Orchitis.** This condition results in inflammation of the testicles and can be caused by a virus or bacteria. Testicular inflammation of this kind is typically associated with mumps. And this may result in long-term testicular damage. I have seen several instances of men who have had mumps in the past and later in life suffered from low testosterone. Whether mumps was a deciding factor is hard to say; however, there does appear to be a correlation in many cases.

- **Prescription drugs.** Pain management is a massive public health issue that costs society an estimated $500 billion

96   Justin Wagner, Joshua R. Dusick, David L. McArthur, Pejman Cohan, Christina Wang, Ronald Swerdloff, W. John Boscardin, and Daniel F. Kelly, "Acute Gonadotroph and Somatotroph Hormonal Suppression after Traumatic Brain Injury," *J Neurotrauma*, 2010 Jun, 27(6): 1007–1019, doi: 10.1089/neu.2009.1092.

annually with numerous prescription drugs dished out by physicians to combat it. Opioids are painkiller drugs widely used to treat moderate to severe pain. Types of opioids include: fentanyl, codeine, morphine, and oxycodone. Research suggests long-term use of opioids can suppress the release of gonadotropins and result in low testosterone. For patients who rely on opioids to treat chronic pain, testosterone replacement appears to be the only solution. However, the best option is to try and wean patients off the medication first because cessation of the drugs appears to reverse the symptoms of hypogonadism.[97]

SSRIs (selective serotonin reuptake inhibitors) are another form of prescription drug that can potentially affect sex hormone concentrations. Examples include citalopram, fluoxetine (Prozac), and paroxetine. One study looked at the effect of SSRIs on testicular tissue versus control groups in 40 male rats. The researchers noted testosterone levels were lower in all groups compared with control groups, suggesting further randomized controlled studies were required to establish their effects. My personal observation is that SSRIs can elevate prolactin levels, with numerous studies appearing to corroborate this.[98,99]

97   Jeffrey A. Gudin, MD Adam Laitman Srinivas Nalamachu, MD, "Opioid Related Endocrinopathy," *Pain Medicine,* Volume 16, Issue suppl_1, 1 October 2015: S9–S15, https://doi.org/10.1111/pme.12926.

98   Young-Min Park, "Serum Prolactin Levels in Patients with Major Depressive Disorder Receiving Selective Serotonin-Reuptake Inhibitor Monotherapy for 3 Months: A Prospective Study," *Psychiatry Investig,* 2017 May, 14(3): 368–371, published online 2017 May 16, doi: 10.4306/pi.2017.14.3.368.

99   P.J. Cowen, P.A. Sargent, "Changes in plasma prolactin during SSRI treatment: evidence for a delayed increase in 5-HT neurotransmission," *Journal of Pharmacology,* July 1, 1997, research article, https://doi.org/10.1177/026988119701100410.

- **Recreational drugs.** There are going to be side effects with any class of drug, and the same applies when it comes to recreational or street drugs. Heroin and morphine are part of the opioid class of drugs and have a similar suppressive effect on testosterone levels. In both human and animal studies, cocaine use can result in disruption of normal testosterone production.[100] Marijuana is seen as relatively innocuous in comparison to "harder" drugs such as cocaine. However, long-term use is associated with lower sex hormone production and lower fertility levels, with one of the primary causes appearing to be from elevated free estrogen levels.

  This is further illustrated by a Danish study on 1,215 men age 18–29, which looked at the association between male hormones, semen quality, and marijuana. The study drew data from men who attended a compulsory medical examination to determine their fitness for military service. The researchers noted that regular marijuana use was *significantly* correlated with lower sperm count.

  Interestingly, marijuana was associated with higher total and free testosterone, although it's not clear whether this was due to tobacco or marijuana.[101] And definitely DO NOT go away thinking that marijuana will boost your testosterone

100   Todd T. Brown, Amy B. Wisniewski, and Adrian S. Dobs, "Gonadal and Adrenal Abnormalities in Drug Users: Cause or Consequence of Drug Use Behavior and Poor Health Outcomes," *Am J Infect Dis*, author manuscript, available in PMC 2007 Mar 15, published in final edited form as: *Am J Infect Dis*, 2006, 2(3): 130–135.

101   Tina Djernis Gundersen, Niels Jørgensen, Anna-Maria Andersson, Anne Kirstine Bang, Loa Nordkap, Niels E. Skakkebæk, Lærke Priskorn, Anders Juul, Tina Kold Jensen, "Association Between Use of Marijuana and Male Reproductive Hormones and Semen Quality: A Study Among 1,215 Healthy Young Men," *American Journal of Epidemiology*, Volume 182, Issue 6, 15 September 2015: 473–481, https://doi.org/10.1093/aje/kwv135.

because the underlying mechanism is not clear. That being said, marijuana appears to have many therapeutic applications, namely in pain management and in cancer treatment. More recently, an extract of marijuana and hemp plant, known as CBD oil, has gained popularity for its purported ability to treat pain and reduce inflammation.

## THE NEXT STEPS

I don't advocate you systematically test every single item on this list to see if it's the cause of your low testosterone. That would be a waste of both time and resources. Instead, look for specific clues from your symptoms and the conditions I've described to help you discern the root cause of your low testosterone. Once you understand the problem, you can attempt to fix it.

There may be instances where the cause is not immediately apparent. Indeed, there may be no clear solution to improve the patient's hormonal profile without medical intervention. If you fail to raise your testosterone despite leading a healthy lifestyle, it's likely you need exogenous testosterone, either in the form of an injectable or cream. That is where the expertise and knowledge of a physician who specializes in hormone balance comes in. This will be discussed in depth in the chapter Testosterone Replacement Therapy Protocols.

However, I want to stress one major thing at this point: Taking testosterone should be your LAST RESORT. Exhaust all other options first.

# CHAPTER 6

# ENDOCRINE DISRUPTORS: OUR BODIES UNDER SIEGE

People are becoming more aware of the damaging effect environmental chemicals and toxins have on our bodies. These are known as "endocrine disruptors" and can be defined as: "substances in our environment, food, and consumer products that interfere with hormone biosynthesis, metabolism, or action resulting in a deviation from normal homeostatic control or reproduction."[102] In other words, they interfere with hormone production—especially testosterone.

Examples of endocrine disruptors include plastics, pesticides, fungicides, and pharmaceutical agents. They can be found in everyday items such as plastic bottles, food cans, detergents, cosmetics, and food additives.[103] This issue has still not received mainstream recognition, or perhaps most people prefer not to acknowledge the situation—that consumerism is making them seriously ill. I suspect it's a combination of both.

We know how important nutrition and exercise are, but rarely, if ever, do we hear about endocrine disruptors. Although given the damage they do to men's health, we should hear about them more often. In recent years, there has been a stark decline in semen quality

---

102   Evanthia Diamanti-Kandarakis, Jean-Pierre Bourguignon, Linda C. Giudice, Russ Hauser, Gail S. Prins, Ana M. Soto, R. Thomas Zoeller, and Andrea C. Gore, "Endocrine-Disrupting Chemicals: An Endocrine Society Scientific Statement," *Endocr Rev*, 2009 Jun, 30(4): 293–342, doi: 10.1210/er.2009-0002.

103   Thaddeus T. Schug, Amanda Janesick, Bruce Blumberg and Jerrold J. Heindel, "Endocrine Disrupting Chemicals and Disease Susceptibility," *J Steroid Biochem Mol Biol*, 2011 Nov, 127(3–5): 204–215, published online 2011 Aug 27, doi: 10.1016/j.jsbmb.2011.08.007.

and testosterone levels, in addition to an increase in testicular cancer among the adult male population.[104] But while researchers scratch their heads searching for a "hypothesis," the reality is that endocrine disruptors are a huge contributor.

Endocrine disruptors are very harmful, so it's important to recognize them to minimize your exposure. Forewarned is forearmed. Although, even if you do everything in your power to avoid them, there is only so much you can do; it's virtually impossible to avoid endocrine disruptors in modern life. In this chapter we will focus on the main ones. And at the end of the chapter, I will present what I believe to be the only real option in the face of this relentless chemical onslaught.

## PLASTICS

Plastics are derived from organic materials such as cellulose, coal, natural gas, salt, and crude oil. In order to create plastic, these materials are refined and synthesized through two main processes: polymerization and polycondensation. Today, there are over 20 different types of plastics in use worldwide.[105]

Over the past century, plastics have become an integral part of our lives. In fact, plastics have become so ubiquitous and indispensable that we no longer imagine life without them. In the medical industry alone, they account for 85% of all medical equipment. They are versatile, cheap to manufacture, and require less energy to produce than alternatives.[106] However, this versatility comes at a steep cost.

---

104   Hueiwang Anna Jeng, "Exposure to Endocrine Disrupting Chemicals and Male Reproductive Health," *Front Public Health,* 2014, 2: 55, published online 2014 Jun 5, prepublished online 2014 Apr 6.

105   Emily J. North and Rolf U. Halden, "Plastics and Environmental Health: The Road Ahead," *Rev Environ Health,* 2013, 28(1): 1–8, doi: 10.1515/reveh-2012-0030.

106   Emily J. Northand, "Plastics. "

Plastics are not only detrimental to the environment, but they are also bad for human health.

Bisphenol A or BPA is a common form of plastic typically used in food and beverage packaging and is one of the most widely produced chemicals worldwide.[107] Our exposure to BPAs is primarily through ingesting contaminated food exposed to plastic.[108] Research classifies BPA as a xenoestrogen that mimics the effects of estradiol in the body. A 2008 study concluded that by mimicking estrogenic activity, BPA causes hyperactivity, attention deficit, and a predisposition to drugs.[109] No wonder Millennials are all over the place. And along with smartphones and technology, this may explain the fragmented attention spans of many young people today.

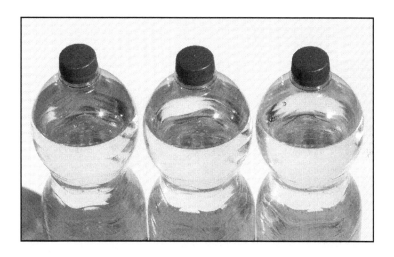

---

107   Rubin BS, "Bisphenol A: an endocrine disruptor with widespread exposure and multiple effects," *J Steroid Biochem Mol Biol,* 2011 Oct, 127(1–2): 27–34, doi: 10.1016/j.jsbmb.2011.05.002.

108   Jeong-HunKanga, Fusao Kondob, Yoshiki Katayamaa, "Human exposure to bisphenol A," *Toxicology,* Volume 226, Issues 2–3, 21 September 2006: 79–89.

109   Douglas C.Jones, Gary W.Miller, "The effects of environmental neurotoxicants on the dopaminergic system: A possible role in drug addiction," *Biochemical Pharmacology,* Volume 76, Issue 5, 1 September 2008: 569–581, https://doi.org/10.1016/j.bcp.2008.05.010.

BPAs have been shown in both human and animal studies to be toxic to Leydig cells (i.e., the cells responsible for producing testosterone in testes), and lower serum testosterone concentrations.[110,111,112] There is evidence correlating body mass index (BMI) and BPA levels,[113] suggesting BPA exposure also plays a key role in the obesity crisis. This makes sense, given obesity is characterized by estrogen dominance.

As a result of the research on BPAs, many manufacturers have come up with BPA-free alternatives for people who want to avoid the harmful effects of BPAs. These alternatives include acrylic, polystyrene, polyethersulfone, and Tritan™. On the surface, it appears to be a novel idea. However, closer inspection reveals BPA-free products are just as bad as their BPA counterparts. One study tested a range of BPA-free alternatives, concluding they were less than safe and actually promoted estrogenic activity in a similar manner to BPAs.[114] Excessive estrogen is bad because it blocks the secretion

---

110 Zhou Q, Miao M, Ran M, Ding L, Bai L, Wu T, Yuan W, Gao E, Wang J, Li G, Li DK, "Serum bisphenol-A concentration and sex hormone levels in men," *Fertil Steril,* 2013 Aug, 100(2): 478–82, doi: 10.1016/j.fertnstert.2013.04.017.

111 Tohei A, Suda S, Taya K, Hashimoto T, Kogo H, "Bisphenol A inhibits testicular functions and increases luteinizing hormone secretion in adult male rats," *Exp Biol Med* (Maywood), 2001 Mar, 226(3): 216–21.

112 Gonçalves GD, Semprebon SC, Biazi BI, Mantovani MS, Fernandes GSA, "Bisphenol A reduces testosterone production in TM3 Leydig cells independently of its effects on cell death and mitochondrial membrane potential," *Reprod Toxicol,* 2018 Mar, 76: 26–34, doi: 10.1016/j.reprotox.2017.12.002.

113 Zhou Q, "The Association between Exposure to Environmental Bisphenol A and Gonadotropic Hormone Levels among Men," *PLoS One,* 2017, 12(1): e0169217, published online 2017 Jan 13, doi: 10.1371/journal.pone.0169217.

114 Bittner GD, Yang CZ, Stoner MA, "Estrogenic chemicals often leach from BPA-free plastic products that are replacements for BPA-containing polycarbonate products," *Environ Health,* 2014 May 28, 13(1): 41, doi: 10.1186/1476-069X-13-41.

of luteinizing hormone, thereby preventing testosterone production, and can even inhibit the production of testosterone in the testes.[115]

## THE WATER SUPPLY

In developed countries, many drink tap water at home, considering it to be safe. The water supply is derived from springs, wells, lakes, rivers, and reservoirs.[116] It typically undergoes cleaning treatment to remove harmful toxins. However, despite these cleaning processes, endocrine disrupting agents can be still be found, particularly in countries such as the US, UK, and Canada. One of the most polarizing and controversial of them all is fluoride.

The United States was one of the first countries to introduce fluoride into the water supply. The main premise for this was to prevent dental decay. Around 5% of the world's population [i.e., 350 million people–including 200 million Americans] drinks artificially fluoridated water. Yet the actual data on whether it prevents dental decay is conflicting. It appears fluoride's main benefit is through topical application (i.e., applying it to the teeth) rather than ingesting it. Countries such as Sweden and Germany have now stopped fluoridating the water supply due to safety concerns.[117]

The 1950s measure to cure dental decay no longer stands up to

115   C.Frye et al., "Endocrine Disrupters: A Review Of Some Sources, Effects, And Mechanisms Of Actions On Behavior And Neuroendocrine Systems," *J Neuroendocrinol*, 2012 Jan, 24(1): 144–159, doi: 10.1111/j.1365-2826.2011.02229.x.

116   O. De Giglio, A. Quaranta, G. Lovero, G. Caggiano, M.T. Montagna, "Mineral water or tap water? An endless debate," *Department of Biomedical Sciences and Human Oncology*, University of Bari Aldo Moro, Italy Ann Ig 2015, 27: 58–65, doi:10.7416/ai.2015.2023.

117   Stephen Peckham and Niyi Awofeso, "Water Fluoridation: A Critical Review of the Physiological Effects of Ingested Fluoride as a Public Health Intervention," *ScientificWorldJournal*, 2014: 293019, published online 2014 Feb 26, doi: 10.1155/2014/293019.

scrutiny, and fluoride exposure can be detrimental to human health. Several animal studies show fluoride reduces testosterone and testicular zinc levels and directly inhibits androgen receptors in the testes.[118] One study in China of male farmers age 18–55 investigated whether fluoride exposure affected serum testosterone and androgen binding proteins (e.g., SHBG). The farmers resided in villages with high fluoride exposure from drinking water versus control groups. The researchers noted lower testosterone levels in the high fluoride group versus the low fluoride group. They concluded men age 18–29 and 30–39 were most susceptible and likely to have lower T when exposed to high fluoride levels.[119]

Another Chinese study looked into the effect of fluoride on the hypothalamic pituitary testicular axis (HPTA) (i.e., testosterone production). They found that higher levels of luteinizing hormone (LH) and lower serum testosterone levels coincided with fluoride-polluted areas. The results point to primary hypogonadism (i.e., failure of the testes to produce testosterone) in these men, where the brain keeps sending a signal to the testes, but there is no response.

The West doesn't have fluoride pollution to the extent that China does, but it's clear that the effects of fluoride can be catastrophic to the male endocrine system. But that's not all. Studies show it can also lower your IQ. One meta study of 27 research papers found that children living in high fluoride exposure areas had lower IQs than

118   Naresh Kumar, Sushma Sood, B Arora, Manjeet Singh, and Beena, "Effect of duration of fluoride exposure on the reproductive system in male rabbits," *J Hum Reprod Sci*, 2010 Sep–Dec, 3(3): 148–152, doi: 10.4103/0974-1208.74159.

119   Duan L, Zhu J, Wang K, Zhou G, Yang Y, Cui L1, Huang H1, Cheng X, Ba Y, "Does Fluoride Affect Serum Testosterone and Androgen Binding Protein with Age-Specificity? A Population-Based Cross-Sectional Study in Chinese Male Farmers," *Biol Trace Elem Res*, 2016 Dec, 174(2): 294–299, epub 2016 May 6.

those in lower exposure or control areas![120] Correlation does not always equal causation, but this is worrying indeed.

## TOXIC FOOD

In order to be grown year-round and resistant to insects and pests, many foods are grown using genetically modified (GMO) seed technology and treated with inordinate amounts of pesticides. This is understandable because farmers want to maintain their crop yield and protect their livelihood. However, using pesticides comes at a cost to the consumer because of their effect on human health. But this is nothing new.

Since 2000, several studies reveal pesticides negatively affect human sperm production and result in poor semen quality.[121] One study at an American infertility clinic measured the reproductive hormones of 238 men against exposure to common insecticides. They found an association between reduction in serum testosterone and exposure to insecticides. The highest exposure to insecticides was associated with a 83 ng/dL (3.0 nmol/L) decline in serum testosterone.[122] That's a big deal. Multiple studies of workers with exposure to pesticides show significant associations between exposure to pesticides and

---

120    Anna L. Choi, Guifan Sun, Ying Zhang, and Philippe Grandjean, "Developmental Fluoride Neurotoxicity: A Systematic Review and Meta-Analysis," *Environ Health Perspect*, 2012 Oct, 120(10): 1362–1368, published online 2012 Jul 20, doi: 10.1289/ehp.1104912.

121    Wissem Mnif, Aziza Ibn Hadj Hassine, Aicha Bouaziz, Aghleb Bartegi, Olivier Thomas, and Benoit Roig, "Effect of Endocrine Disruptor Pesticides: A Review," *Int J Environ Res Public Health*, 2011 Jun, 8(6): 2265–2303, published online 2011 Jun 17, doi: 10.3390/ijerph8062265.

122    Meeker JD, Ryan L, Barr DB, Hauser R, "Exposure to nonpersistent insecticides and male reproductive hormones," *Epidemiology*, 2006 Jan, 17(1): 61–8.

lowering of male sex hormones.[123,124,125] Clearly, chronic low-level exposure is not good for your health.

One study looked at the relationship between fatty acid intake, male reproductive hormones, and testicular volume (i.e., size of the testes) and found a positive correlation between intake of omega-6 fatty acids (proinflammatory) and higher luteinizing hormone levels (LH). These results suggest these fats negatively affect testicular function.[126] The researchers also found trans fat intake associated with lower sperm.[127]

If processed foods weren't already bad enough, evidence suggests they also act as endocrine disruptors. One processed food ingredient that is ubiquitous today is soy. Soy additives are found in meats, sausages, pasta, and breakfast cereals. One Finnish study investigated if food packaging was responsible for contaminating food and

123   Manfo FP, Moundipa PF, Déchaud H, Tchana AN, Nantia EA, Zabot MT, Pugeat M, "Effect of agropesticides use on male reproductive function: a study on farmers in Djutitsa (Cameroon)," *Environ Toxicol,* 2012 Jul, 27(7): 423–32, doi: 10.1002/tox.20656. Epub 2010 Nov 29.

124   Mehrpour O, Karrari P, Zamani N, Tsatsakis AM, Abdollahi M, "Occupational exposure to pesticides and consequences on male semen and fertility: a review," *Toxicol Lett,* 2014 Oct 15, 230(2): 146–56, doi: 10.1016/j.toxlet.2014.01.029. Epub 2014 Jan 30.

125   Panuwet P et al., "Investigation of associations between exposures to pesticides and testosterone levels in Thai farmers," *Arch Environ Occup Health,* 2017 Sep 13:1–14, doi: 10.1080/19338244.2017.1378606.

126   Lidia Mínguez Alarcón, Jorge E Chavarro, Jaime Mendiola, Manuela Roca, Cigdem Tanrikut, Jesús Vioque, Niels Jørgensen, and Alberto M TorresCantero, "Fatty acid intake in relation to reproductive hormones and testicular volume among healthy young men," *Asian J Androl,* 2017 Mar–Apr, 19(2): 184–190, published online 2016 Oct 28, doi: 10.4103/1008682X. 190323.

127   Jorge E. Chavarro, Lidia Mínguez-Alarcón, Jaime Mendiola, Ana Cutillas-Tolín, José J. López-Espín, and Alberto M. Torres-Cantero, "*Trans* fatty acid intake is inversely related to total sperm count in young healthy men," *Hum Reprod,* 2014 Mar, 29(3): 429–440, published online 2014 Jan 12, doi: 10.1093/humrep/det464.

promoting estrogenic activity, or whether food inside the packaging caused estrogenic activity. Most food wrappers and foods tested did not cause significant estrogenic activity. However, researchers discovered industrially prepared hamburgers and salami containing soy were "highly estrogenic."[128] Therefore, it's highly likely other foods containing soy ingredients will have the same effect.

## THE AIR WE BREATHE

Studies show inhalation of *indoor* dust may be comparable to food in terms of endocrine disruption. Endocrine disrupting chemicals are found in household products, building materials, household appliances, furniture, and carpets. These substances contribute to indoor dust—a mixture of organic and inorganic compounds. Carpets are one of the biggest repositories for dust,[129] and of all the chemicals found in dust, phthalate is one of the most common. Phthalates are used primarily as plasticizers to coat plastics. They can also be found in pills, detergents, food products, and packaging. A large-scale study of over 2,000 people linked phthalates with a 24–34.1% drop in testosterone levels among young boys age 6–12 years,[130] so imagine what it's like with adults who've been exposed to them for years.

---

128    Omoruyi IM, Kabiersch G, Pohjanvirta R, "Commercial processed food may have endocrine-disrupting potential: soy-based ingredients making the difference," *Food Addit Contam Part A Chem Anal Control Expo Risk Assess*, 2013, 30(10): 1722–7, doi: 10.1080/19440049.2013.817025.

129    Hyun-Min Hwang, Eun-Kee Park, Thomas M. Young, and Bruce D. Hammock, "Occurrence of endocrine-disrupting chemicals in indoor dust," *Sci Total Environ*, 2008 Oct 1, 404(1): 26–35, published online 2008 Jul 15, doi: 10.1016/j.scitenv.2008.05.031.

130    John D. Meeker, Kelly K. Ferguson, "Urinary Phthalate Metabolites Are Associated With Decreased Serum Testosterone in Men, Women, and Children From NHANES 2011–2012," *The Journal of Clinical Endocrinology & Metabolism*, 2014, jc.2014-2555, DOI: 10.1210/jc.2014-2555.

We are also exposed to endocrine disruptors when we go outside. One study looked at the effect of jet fuel exposure on multiple generations of rats, and the results were frightening. It concluded jet fuel exposure promotes "transgenerational inheritance of disease." In other words, disease is passed down. They also found environmental exposures to it resulted in sperm mutations in later generations of rats.[131] In another study, adult male rats were exposed to low-level diesel exhaust fumes, and fetuses suffered from an "irreversible decrease in daily sperm production."[132] While our exposure to these substances is at a low level, it all adds up.

## DIRTY ELECTRICITY

In his book, *Dirty Electricity: Electrification and the Diseases of Civilization*, Dr. Sam Milham warns us about the health dangers posed by dirty electricity and electromagnetic interference (EMI). After more than 50 years as a physician and epidemiologist (someone who studies the incidence and distribution of disease), Milham concluded the electrification of society (i.e., introduction of electricity) was primarily responsible for so-called "civilization diseases." These include heart disease, cancer, diabetes, and even suicide.

Milham uses historical data from the United States to demonstrate the effect electrification had on society. For example, if you lived in New York in the early 1900s, your average life expectancy was into the low-50s. But if you were Amish or lived in rural Mississippi or rural New York, your average life expectancy went into the 70s. The

131   Rebecca Tracey, Mohan Manikkam, Carlos Guerrero-Bosagna, and Michael K. Skinne. "Hydrocarbons (Jet Fuel JP-8) Induce Epigenetic Transgenerational Inheritance of Obesity, Reproductive Disease and Sperm Epimutations," *Reprod Toxicol,* 2013 Apr, 36: 104–116, published online 2013 Jan 25, doi: 10.1016/j.reprotox.2012.11.011.

132   Takeda K, Tsukue N, Yoshida S, "Endocrine-disrupting activity of chemicals in diesel exhaust and diesel exhaust particles," *Environ Sci,* 2004,11(1): 33–45.

difference between the two areas? New York was electrified; the rural areas were not. After looking at data from the 1930s, he notes urban cancer mortality was 50% to 80% higher than in rural areas. He goes on to say that chronic EMI exposure increases your risk for cancer, citing an example of a breast cancer epidemic among staff at a school with a cell tower on campus.

This led me to investigate whether the technology we use today causes endocrine disruption. What about cell phones? We all have one; we sleep next to them and carry them around all day. In short, we can't live without them. One study of 153 men in a fertility clinic in the United States found no association between cell phone use and sperm quality.[133] Another study investigated the effect of electromagnetic radiation from cell phones on rats. The researchers observed that LH, FSH, and serum testosterone decreased significantly in rats exposed to the radiation versus control groups. They concluded chronic exposure to cell phone radiation leads to reduced testicular function.[134] A separate study found a correlation between cell phone exposure, DNA fragmentation (i.e., abnormal sperm), and sperm motility (i.e., ability of the sperm to move).[135]

Wi-Fi is a common electromagnetic frequency (EMF) that we are exposed to daily. There are few studies on the effect of Wi-Fi on human male testicular function, but the available data is alarming. It's led some authors to call it, "an uncontrolled global experiment on

---

133    Ryan C. Lewis, Ph.D. et al., "Self-reported mobile phone use and semen parameters among men from a fertility clinic," *Reprod Toxicol*, 2017 Jan, 67: 42–47, published online 2016 Nov 9, doi: 10.1016/j.reprotox.2016.11.008.

134    Oyewopo AO, Olaniyi SK, Oyewopo CI, Jimoh AT, "Radiofrequency electromagnetic radiation from cell phone causes defective testicular function in male Wistar rats," *J Urol*, 2007 Jan, 177(1): 395–9.

135    Igor Gorpinchenko, Oleg Nikitin, Oleg Banyra, and Alexander Shulyak, "The influence of direct mobile phone radiation on sperm quality," *Cent European J Urol*, 2014, 67(1): 65–71, published online 2014 Apr 17, doi: 10.5173/ceju.2014.01.art14.

the health of mankind."[136] One study investigated the link between sperm motility and laptop computers connected to the Internet via Wi-Fi. Sperm samples were taken from 29 healthy donors and split into two groups. One was used as a control, while the other group was exposed to a wireless Internet connected laptop for four hours. The researchers found that sperm exposed to Wi-Fi had a significant decrease in motility and increase in DNA fragmentation.[137] Another study on 16 adult male rats investigated whether exposure to a 2.4 GHz Wi-Fi frequency (the most common frequency) could cause DNA damage to organ tissues. The study concluded long-term Wi-Fi exposure did not cause DNA damage to organ tissues but did cause damage the DNA of the rat testes,[138] suggesting the testes are more sensitive than other organs to radio frequencies.

There is one more study that demonstrates the harmful effects of Wi-Fi; while it was not overly scientific, the results are fascinating. A group of schoolgirls from Denmark took 400 seeds of watercress and placed them in 12 trays. They placed six trays in two separate rooms at room temperature. For 12 days, both sets of trays got the same amount of sun and water, while six trays were exposed to Wi-Fi routers. The result? The seeds without exposure to the router grew as normal, but those next to the router did not grow—and some even

---

136    Markov M, Grigoriev YG, "Wi-Fi technology—an uncontrolled global experiment on the health of mankind," *Electromagn Biol Med*, 2013 Jun, 32(2): 200–8, doi: 10.3109/15368378.2013.776430.

137    Avendaño C, Mata A, Sanchez Sarmiento CA, Doncel GF, "Use of laptop computers connected to internet through Wi-Fi decreases human sperm motility and increases sperm DNA fragmentation," *Fertil Steril*, 2012 Jan, 97(1): 39–45.e2, doi: 10.1016/j.fertnstert.2011.10.012.

138    Akdag MZ, Dasdag S, Canturk F, Karabulut D, Caner Y, Adalier N, "Does prolonged radiofrequency radiation emitted from Wi-Fi devices induce DNA damage in various tissues of rats?" *J Chem Neuroanat*, 2016 Sep, 75(Pt B): 116–22, doi: 10.1016/j.jchemneu.2016.01.003.

died![139] Wi-Fi has become indispensable to us; however, it appears we still do not fully appreciate the implications to human health.

## HOW TO AVOID ENDOCRINE DISRUPTORS

So what can you do to avoid endocrine disruptors? If it's not already apparent, it's next to impossible to avoid endocrine disruptors unless you live in a cave. In fact, you can live in the Arctic Circle and still not be immune! Studies in Greenland show more girls than boys are born because of exposure to man-made chemicals.[140]

However, there are things you can do to minimize exposure to endocrine disruptors. You can try to avoid plastics, but it's difficult to avoid them altogether. Personally, I use stainless steel containers for protein shakes, and glass containers for meals. Where possible, you should replace plastic containers with glass or stainless steel, and the quality is better and they last longer. Although, even these items still have a plastic component. And as we've seen, BPA-free alternatives aren't much use either.

To avoid endocrine disruptors, I believe in striking a happy medium. Minimize plastic exposure, but don't let it rule your life. There is a tendency in the health space to go overboard with this stuff and become obsessed. **A healthy lifestyle should improve your quality of life—not become your ENTIRE existence.** If I'm outside and I'm thirsty, then I'll buy a bottle of water whether it's plastic or not. I won't spend hours looking for a store that sells glass bottles.

---

139  "Wifi Experiment Done By A Group Of 9th Grade Students Got Serious International Attention. THIS Is Why ..." Outside the Box, accessed November 29, 2018, http://ofthebox.org/wifi-experiment-done-group-9th-grade-students-got-serious-international-attention/.

140  "Health effects associated with lifestyle, diet and exposure to PTS," https://www.loe.org/images/content/080725/Health%20Effects%20of%20POPs%20in%20Arctic.pdf.

When it comes to drinking water, you have two options: You can buy a water filter for your home. They are cost effective and remove most impurities, but they won't get rid of things like fluoride. For that you will need a professional water filter you attach to the tap. The water goes through the machine, and the fluoride is filtered out. A machine like this may cost several hundred dollars, but it will eventually pay for itself with the money you save buying bottled water. Remember, health is an investment. You can buy plastic bottles if you don't want to drink out of the tap, but then the issue becomes the contamination of the water with xenoestrogens.[141]

So how do you limit your exposure to endocrine disruptors in the air? Prevent dust particles from accumulating in your home by vacuuming and cleaning regularly. That comes with its own hazards, though, as most household cleaning products contain a glut of toxic chemicals. In the US, some household products have the "Safer Choice" label on them. The Environmental Protection Agency gives products this label when they pass strict human health and environmental criteria.[142] See if there is something similar in your country.

Avoiding endocrine disruptors in foods is straightforward. **The simple method is: DON'T EAT CRAP.** Most of your food should come from natural, non-processed sources anyway (i.e., chicken, fruit, vegetables, etc.). Aim to eat organic where possible and avoid eating meat from animals raised with synthetic hormones. Once again, I don't believe in living like a monk. We're only human, after all. That's why I abide by the 80/20 rule. If you eat clean most of the week and at the weekend you feel like a little treat, go right ahead.

---

141  Wagner M, Oehlmann J., "Endocrine disruptors in bottled mineral water: total estrogenic burden and migration from plastic bottles," *Environ Health Perspect*, 2009 Jun, 117(6): A241.

142  "Frequently Asked Questions on Safer Choice," United States Environmental Protection Agency, accessed November 29, 2018, https://www.epa.gov/saferchoice/frequently-asked-questions-safer-choice.

The biggest challenge is technology. We're connected 24/7 and spend countless hours glued to our smartphones. And as we're so dependent on them, calls to limit time on electronic devices will fall on deaf ears. Therefore, I recommend minimizing exposure to harmful radio waves from cell phones by putting them in airplane mode whenever you can. Why do you always need to be available anyway? Some downtime from technology is good for you. Aim to keep electronic devices out of your bedroom, especially at night. This will minimize exposure to harmful chemicals. But be under no illusion; trying to avoid them amounts to a drop in the ocean. We are bombarded daily by low-level endocrine disrupting chemicals. Even if you try and avoid them, they will affect you anyway.

# CHAPTER 7

# YOUNG MEN AND THE ANABOLIC STEROID EPIDEMIC

In the opening chapter we discussed the low-testosterone epidemic affecting men of all ages. We've seen how environmental and cultural factors have conspired to create this epidemic. But aside from environmental and lifestyle factors, there is something else contributing to the low testosterone epidemic. That is anabolic and androgenic steroid (AAS) abuse. I believe it to be such a big problem that it will become an epidemic in itself, so I've devoted an entire chapter to the topic. Some researchers suggest AAS abuse may even be the most common cause of hypogonadism in young men.[143]

There are several reasons why widespread AAS abuse remains under the radar. First, the possession of anabolic steroids is illegal in many countries, so people taking them aren't exactly going to advertise it. Furthermore, because it's illegal, no official figures exist for how many people take AAS. So unless you are in the "scene," you would have no idea this problem exists.

My eyes were opened after consulting daily with young men who abused anabolic steroids. And they all typically had one thing in common: Low testosterone. After a cycle of steroids (sometimes several), their natural testosterone production was in the gutter. In many cases, the damage was irreversible. And I've seen countless young men with testosterone levels of men three times their age.

When I was younger, all I knew about AAS was that taking them

---

143    Coward RM et al., "Anabolic steroid induced hypogonadism in young men," *J Urol*, 2013 Dec, 190(6): 2200–5, doi: 10.1016/j.juro.2013.06.010.

could damage my health, which was enough to deter me. Unfortunately, many men show no fear of the damaging effects. In this chapter, we'll look at the consequences of taking anabolic steroids and what motivates young men to use them. We'll also separate fact from fiction about steroid cycles.

## A BRIEF HISTORY OF ANABOLIC STEROIDS

For centuries, human beings have recognized the muscle-building and invigorating power of the male testes. Of course, they didn't realize it was testosterone primarily responsible for these effects. Even in 1400 BC, Ayurveda, an ancient Indian system of medicine, recommended testicular tissue as a cure for impotence. It wasn't until the 19th century, though, that things progressed further, when Charles-Edouard Brown-Séquard injected himself with a subcutaneous "liquid obtained from the testicles of animals." As a result, he reported improvements in physical strength and appetite.[144] And in 1935, Adolf Butenandt and Leopold Ruzicka finally managed to chemically isolate and synthesize testosterone.

After the discovery of testosterone, people began to modify testosterone and other androgens (e.g., dihydrotestosterone), to produce synthetic drugs emphasizing anabolic properties. At this point, people outside the academic world became interested. Subsequently, competitive bodybuilders began to use anabolics as a way to increase muscle mass and gain an edge in competition. This practice began to filter down to regular gym-goers who wanted to gain more muscle. Fast-forward to today; anabolic steroids can be bought and sold at many gyms.

---

144   Brown-Séquard C.E., "The effects produced on man by subcutaneous injection of a liquid obtained from the testicles of animals," *Lancet* (1889) 137: 105–107.

## WHY DO YOUNG MEN TAKE ANABOLIC STEROIDS?

Young men do not take AAS in droves to gain muscle for the hell of it. There is clearly an evolutionary component involved. A man with a muscular physique is attractive to women because, among other things, muscle tone signals dominance, strength, and security. Subconsciously, muscularity also represents traits such as discipline, mental fortitude, and tenacity. You probably don't need me to tell you men want to build muscle to appear more attractive to women—but that's not all there is to it.

In a society hooked on instant gratification, young men are seduced by the promise of a quick fix; steroids can offer muscle gain in a short time. Many men are deluded into believing they can take shortcuts on almost anything. Why bust your ass for years in the gym, create the right habits, eat the right foods, and postpone gratification when you can do it in a few months? But as we'll see shortly, shortcuts have consequences.

Our Western way of thinking places emphasis on an external versus an internal locus of control. This means we always look for solutions outside of ourselves. This is reflected in Western medicine where drugs and treatment are the main focus to fight disease. And hence why men look to anabolics for a solution to their problem.

And it's not just women who feel pressure from society to look a certain way. Men feel it too. In particular, social media has created a totally unrealistic ideal for men to live up to. They see pictures of six-pack abs on Instagram and feel inadequate, so they look to AAS to fill the void. But what these young men don't appreciate is that often these pictures are a complete fabrication, and their social media idols will take multiple pictures to get the perfect shot—or use Photoshop—thus creating a distorted reality for their followers.

## THE BRO MENTALITY

The most troubling aspect of AAS abuse among young men is their casual attitude toward it. Perhaps it's the exuberance of youth or lack of life experience, but all too often young men take AAS without considering the consequences. Worse yet, they base their decisions on things they read on a steroid forum or heard from guys at the gym. I call this the "Bro Mentality."

The Bro Mentality is the pursuit of gains at any cost. When you have the Bro Mentality, you are willing to try almost anything, as long as it leads to building muscle. People on forums advocate aggressively stacking multiple steroids in a reckless manner, just for the gains. This mentality is even seen in forums supposedly dedicated to testosterone replacement therapy. After being on prescription testosterone for a few weeks, guys will complain they haven't seen much by the way of gains. They think muscle gains must come immediately, else there's a problem.

Guys are also influenced by their training partners or people they see at the gym. Because these people are muscular and look like they know how to train, it makes an impression on these men. They assume that, because of their size, someone knows what they're talking about, and they're all too willing to take the advice at face value. But there is nothing scientific about these quick-fix methods. The doses used are massive, often without rhyme or reason. And blood tests are not considered, so there's no consciousness of the massive damage being done to the body.

I often wonder how men can make such a weighty decision based on such bad information? If anything, before I began testosterone replacement therapy, I was overcautious. It wasn't until I read several books on it that I felt comfortable to go ahead with treatment.

Nowadays most men don't read or appreciate books. A book takes hours of research and dedication, meaning much thought has gone into it, so its value is considerably higher than a forum post that takes minutes to create. In fact, there is no comparison between the two. But once again, people want to take shortcuts. Google has all the answers!

This Bro Mentality is typified by a conversation I once had with a 28-year-old man during a flight. The conversation began with the normal small talk. When we talked about work, I told him I coach and teach men about health, fitness, and hormone optimization. Subsequently, he confided to me he was planning to do a steroid cycle of boldenone (Equipoise) stacked with testosterone propionate for several weeks, then he would cycle off it with post-cycle therapy (PCT). He was excited about doing a cycle and gaining muscle yet seemed unfazed by the potential consequences.

After he outlined his plan, I asked him some questions. "Have you had a blood test done before to see what your testosterone levels are?" I explained he should at least have a baseline level prior to doing a cycle. Next I asked, "What do you know about these drugs? Is the source reliable?" He admitted he had never taken a blood test and didn't have a clue how any of these drugs worked. And to top it off, he'd convinced himself he was getting the drugs from a good source—from the guys in the gym!

At this point I delivered home truths. I explained even a short cycle could permanently damage his testosterone production. It might not, but that was the risk he was taking. Suddenly, the blood drained from his face, and he stared at me wide-eyed in horror. He lived in fairytale land, where steroids only build muscle and have no consequences. Despite his ignorance, he was willing to play Russian roulette with his body. I find it surreal so many young men are willing to gamble with their health. Yet they believe other people are in harm's way, not them. "It won't happen to me!"

This guy was broad-shouldered and powerful. With a little effort and dedication, he could easily have a quality physique. But he was overweight, and over the course of a two-hour flight he drank several beers. In reality, he had **no business** doing a cycle of steroids. Instead, he should have focused on mastering the basics of proper nutrition and training. Sadly, he was seduced by the quick-fix approach of a steroid cycle. Little did he know it causes more problems than it solves. I gave him my number, inviting him to reach out to me if he needed advice, but he never called.

## STEROID CYCLES: WHAT GOES UP MUST COME DOWN

On paper it seems like a great idea: Do a 12-week cycle, gain muscle, then go on post-cycle therapy (PCT) to restore natural testosterone production. It's not for long, so it can't be that bad right? Wrong. Because once you remove drugs from the equation the gains disappear, **What goes up must come down.**

And the idea you can go on PCT to restart your natural production of testosterone is laughable. Think about it, your natural production has been shut down for weeks, months, or even years in some cases. Your endocrine system has been taken over by an exogenous substance and is probably permanently damaged. Using hCG or Clomid (discussed later) may help for a time, but once again, when you remove the drug, the effect disappears. If you have messed up your body's natural production of testosterone, no amount of PCT is going to save you. Jay Campbell, author of *The Testosterone Optimization Therapy Bible*, explains the myth of the "cycling," and how destructive and pointless it is:

Once you are ON, you do not come OFF. Once you are using, you don't stop using. You can lower your dosage to a TRT dose (i.e., a therapeutic dose) with time, and many guys do this for health reasons, but you can never come off completely (if you want to retain the muscle mass and size gained from using supraphysiologic dosages of AAS).

The idea of "cycling" is a myth. Taking steroids for a "cycle" and never taking them again would be idiotic and pointless, as the positive effects go away completely. What cycling actually means is that you go through periods of higher doses and lower doses (also known as "blasting and cruising"), while taking different compounds at different times. Every steroid user I've known who went completely "cold turkey" has returned to their natural levels of size and strength. **Every single time.145**

Another thing to mention about cycling is weight gain. There is a HUGE difference between gaining scale weight and quality muscle mass. The weight gain on most steroid cycles is not from muscle mass but from increased body fat and water retention. "Bulking" diets, where guys eat everything in sight, usually result in more fat than muscle gain. Water retention also occurs from massive steroid doses. As a result, many guys who cycle end up looking bloated and fat, instead of looking like Greek gods. Hardly worth messing up your endocrine system for.

To illustrate this point further, one study of 61 healthy men 18–35 over 20 weeks measured the effect of various testosterone enanthate injections (20, 50, 125, 300, or 600 mg) on muscle capillaries (i.e., muscle size). Interestingly, the authors did not observe a significant

---

145  Campbell, *The Testosterone Optimization Therapy Bible.*

difference in capillary density between the groups.[146] In other words, it takes time to build quality muscle, and steroid cycles are not going to result in meaningful gains.

## ANABOLIC STEROIDS AND HEALTH

It's not only the short-term cycling mindset that's idiotic, it's also the massive doses of AAS and their impact on health. What you see on the outside is not always a reflection of the inside. So what are the side effects and impact of taking AAS?

- **Elevated estrogen levels.** The word estrogen strikes fear into the hearts of men who take AAS. In men, estrogen is primarily produced through the conversion of testosterone to estradiol. The aromatase enzyme is abundant in adipose (fat) tissue. Estradiol (the main form of estrogen in men) rises with testosterone, and the more testosterone you take, the more estrogen your body will produce.

  You can get unwanted estrogenic side effects by using supraphysiologic (high) doses of AAS. These include puffiness (moon face), water retention, bloating, gynecomastia (bitch tits), poor erection quality, and low sex drive.

- **Hair loss.** It appears that baldness as a result of androgen use is because the individual was already predisposed to hair loss.[147] In other words, if you were already going to lose your hair, taking steroids may speed up the process.

---

146    Sinha-Hikim I. et al., "Testosterone-induced increase in muscle size in healthy young men is associated with muscle fiber hypertrophy," *Am J Physiol Endocrinol Metab*, 2002 Jul, 283(1): E154–64.

147    Jay R. Hoffman and Nicholas A. Ratamess, "Medical Issues Associated with Anabolic Steroid Use: Are They Exaggerated?" *J Sports Sci Med*, 2006 Jun, 5(2): 182–193, published online 2006 Jun 1.

- **Elevated blood pressure.** Anabolic steroids elevate hematocrit levels (a marker to measure total red blood volume versus total volume of blood) and stimulate red blood cell production. In turn, this raises blood pressure and means your heart works harder to pump blood around the body. An overworked and stressed heart is a ticking time bomb.

- **Insomnia.** Taking massive doses of AAS wires your central nervous system (CNS) and keeps you awake at night. This is because AAS act on neurotransmitter pathways, such as serotonin and dopamine that regulate the sleep-wake cycle.[148]

- **Lowered fertility and testosterone levels.** When you use androgens, the body detects increased testosterone levels and stops its own natural production. This results in lowered fertility, if not infertility, for the duration of steroid use—and possibly beyond. Recovery of fertility is possible after cessation of steroids. However, this may take months or years in some cases.[149]

- **Suicide.** This is rare among men who use AAS but worth mentioning. If you're struggling with personal problems in your life, anabolics are not the solution. If anything, they can exacerbate the problem because they can alter your perception of reality. They won't turn you into a nut job because that's not how they work. But at high doses, they can make you more

---

148  Bertozzi G, Sessa F, Albano GD, Sani G, Maglietta F, Roshan MHK, Volti GL, Bernardini R, Avola R, Pomara C, Salerno M., "The Role of Anabolic Androgenic Steroids in Disruption of the Physiological Function in Discrete Areas of the Central Nervous System," *Mol Neurobiol*, 2017 Oct 2, doi: 10.1007/s12035-017-0774-1.

149  J Abram McBride and Robert M Coward, "Recovery of spermatogenesis following testosterone replacement therapy or anabolic-androgenic steroid use," *Asian J Androl*, 2016 May–Jun, 18(3): 373–380, doi: 10.4103/1008-682X.173938.

irritable and emotional, making your problems seem worse than they are.

One study investigated the suicides of eight males ages of 21–33 years with a history of ongoing or discontinued anabolic steroid use. After a psychological autopsy, in all cases they determined "risk factors of suicidality are likely to be independent of the use of AAS were present."[150] In other words, it was not AAS that caused suicide, but they may contribute to feelings of suicide in individuals already predisposed.

If you go off steroids cold turkey, you can suffer withdrawal symptoms and go into depression. This is because your body has shut down its own natural production of testosterone. So it may take several weeks for your body to start producing it again. No testosterone = DEATH—if not physically, then certainly mentally. **Do not put yourself in this position.**

- **Recreational drug use.** It's well established that taking "soft" drugs can be a gateway to harder substances, (e.g., marijuana to cocaine. You might think a cycle of steroids would never lead you to take other drugs. However, the psychological barrier to entry is lowered once you take any type of drug, making you more amenable to experiment.

One interesting study looked at the link between substance abuse and the use of AAS. They studied 223 men receiving treatment for alcohol, cocaine, and opioid abuse. In total, 29 men (13%) reported prior AAS use. The vast majority who used AAS also became opioid dependent. And of the men interviewed in detail, many said they **received opioids from the same person who sold them steroids at the gym.** Among

---

150   Thiblin I, Runeson B, Rajs J., "Anabolic androgenic steroids and suicide," *Ann Clin Psychiatry*, 1999 Dec, 11(4): 223–31.

the steroid users, 75% said it was the first drug they ever injected.[151] That's not to say by virtue of taking steroids you will become a drug addict, but you should be aware of the psychology behind taking drugs.

While there are negative side effects that come with anabolic steroid use, the majority are transient and reversible upon cessation of the drugs.[152] Does this mean the impact of anabolic steroids is purely negative? Few things in life are truly black and white. If they had zero benefits, no one would take them. Here are some of the positive effects of AAS:

- Increased protein synthesis
- Enhanced recovery between workouts
- Increased glycogen storage
- Increased fat-loss (lipolysis)
- Increased strength, power, and lean body mass
- Increased bone mineral density[153]

The benefits of AAS mirror taking therapeutic testosterone. The difference is: One damages your health, while the other promotes it. Regardless of what I write, many will take anabolic steroids anyway. While I don't ever advocate them, if you're going to do it, at least educate yourself. For an excellent primer on AAS, I recommend you read the chapter Anabolic Steroids—the Stone Cold Truth in *The*

---

151   Kanayama G, Cohane GH, Weiss RD, Pope HG, "Past anabolic-androgenic steroid use among men admitted for substance abuse treatment: an underrecognized problem?" *J Clin Psychiatry*, 2003 Feb, 64(2): 156–60.

152   Jay R. Hoffman and Nicholas A. Ratamess, "Medical Issues Associated with Anabolic Steroid Use: Are They Exaggerated?" *J Sports Sci Med*, 2006 Jun, 5(2): 182–193, published online 2006 Jun 1.

153   Jay R. Hoffman and Nicholas A. Ratamess, "Medical Issues Associated with Anabolic Steroid Use: Are They Exaggerated?" *J Sports Sci Med*, 2006 Jun, 5(2): 182–193, published online 2006 Jun 1.

*Testosterone Optimization Therapy Bible* (TOTBible.com).[154] And for further reading, William Llewellyn's *ANABOLICS* is a must.

The takeaway message here is: if you take anabolic steroids, you had better be prepared for the consequences. Otherwise, don't start in the first place.

154   Campbell, *The Testosterone Optimization Therapy Bible.*

# INTERVIEW WITH JIM BROWN

Jim Brown is a former bodybuilder and co-founder of Optimized Life Nutrition (optimizedlifenutrition.com), responsible for industry-leading supplements such as Energy Memory Focus.

Jim is peerless in his knowledge on all things optimization: health, nutrition, training, hormones, and supplementation. This knowledge has been earned through decades of experimentation, study, and coaching elite-level athletes. And I myself have been fortunate enough to receive his wisdom in recent years. So when Jim Brown speaks, you better sit up and listen.

**Daniel Kelly:** Jim, in the past you've said, "Bodybuilding and health don't go in the same sentence." Does this mean bodybuilding and health are mutually exclusive?

**Jim Brown:** I have changed my definition of bodybuilding over the years, but competitive bodybuilding, or even looking as though you compete, has absolutely nothing to do with health and **everything to do with look**. A huge, shredded physique is also a body under massive stress and abuse that will likely have a steep cost.

**Daniel Kelly:** It seems young men will take steroids without the faintest idea what they're doing, or the repercussions involved. Why do you think they feel so compelled, despite the risks?

**Jim Brown:** At the time, the risks seem a long way away. I recall a conversation I once had with Dan Duchaine, and I asked him, "When do I stop?" and he answered, "When you get sick." Fortunately, I was very honest with myself, and knowing when to stop was determined by answering, "How far am I going with this?"

My goal was to be the best bodybuilder I could be after training and competing naturally for 11 years. Then after three years of research, I started using AAS with the intention of using until my body couldn't handle it anymore. At which point, I fully expected to go on TRT for the rest of my life. That decision led to me administering testosterone shots for the last 20 years. So back to the question: Why are these guys compelled? That's easy, to be jacked and shredded, and they think AAS will get them there. The consequences are a long way off, hiding in the fog.

**Daniel Kelly:** The Golden Era of bodybuilding produced guys such as Arnold Schwarzenegger, Mike Mentzer, and Larry Scott. Back then, many used AAS but in conservative doses. However, the approach today is to push the envelope and take massive doses at all costs. Why do you think this is?

**Jim Brown:** Those guys mentioned above would be low-level national competitors nowadays IF that—even in the new Classic Physique Class the NPC has come out with. It's a different game today, but it's a great point. These guys were masters of all aspects of the game and *decided* to use AAS—not the opposite. They produced amazing physiques that were both larger and more extreme than most people realize. You won't appreciate it unless you have been in a room with these jacked dudes.

**Daniel Kelly:** People often confuse TRT with anabolic steroids. What is the difference between them, and why do people confuse the two?

**Jim Brown:** By definition testosterone is an anabolic steroid. Just like a Tesla is a car; there are many cars used for many purposes. Taking hormones in supraphysiological doses is much different than trying to correct a clinical need necessary to optimize health. It is an uneducated, knee-jerk reaction to the word *testosterone*.

**Daniel Kelly:** Young guys resort to AAS primarily to build muscle. Is it possible to build a great physique without resorting to drugs?

**Jim Brown:** Just being "natural" you can build a great physique. Let's get real here. When I lived in Vegas, I would estimate with my expert eye that the rush hour crowd at Gold's Gym contained a very high AAS user to not ratio. I would say as high as 80% of the guys were "on." To the uneducated eye, this ratio was much lower maybe 20%.

There are hordes of guys using anabolics that still look like shit, why? A couple reasons. First, they never mastered their own body—you must master the principles of nutrition and training before even considering AAS. If you start a "cycle" as a fat, chubby-looking dude and have been training for a while, you are just going to be a larger version of that guy at the end of your cycle.

For example, if you're training now but can't seem to figure out how to bring up your chest, a cycle won't change that. My point? You can make massive changes to your body by mastering it with normal levels of hormones.

**Daniel Kelly:** Some bodybuilders believe they can use post-cycle therapy (PCT) to restore their own natural production of testos-terone after AAS. How much of an impact does AAS have on your natural production, and can you really use PCT after a cycle?

**Jim Brown:** "PCT" was an absolute joke to me. I never have been off testosterone with the exception of giving my own body a chance to kick back on after 12 years of massive doses. The whole idea that you are going to use AAS for a few weeks or months then come off, just restart your system, and keep those gains for good with no cost is childish. But that seems to be the dream being sold to the kids these days.

I researched enough back in the day to realize it didn't add up. Anytime you take exogenous testosterone or any other anabolic steroid, your natural production will be negatively affected. Some people can do cycle, and after a period, their testosterone production will come back online.

Now is that to say it's damaged or negatively affected? That is a difficult question to answer with all the variables involved, but the real question I would ask is: What the hell is one or two cycles going to do for you? How long will those changes—if positive—last? How was your body impacted? Did you do blood work pre, during, and after to effectively evaluate if your body is capable of taking AAS without severe negative consequences? Then you must be honest with your risk assessment based on that. And that's before even *considering* family history of cardiac or vascular related conditions.

# CHAPTER 8

## SUPPLEMENTS FOR YOUNG MEN

Most guys have it completely the wrong way around when it comes to supplements. As with the previous chapter on steroids, they look to supplements as some kind of magic bullet. And we all know guys who spend hundreds, if not thousands of dollars on supplements. They are always searching for that ONE supplement, the game changer to transform their workouts and physique. Yet their diet is horrendous, they get minimal sleep, and they rarely train consistently. Once again, these guys need to master the basics before they even think about supplements.

But let's say you've got everything dialed in and you want to take your health to the next level. In that case, you need to take supplements. And as we've seen in previous chapters, you will struggle to get the right amount of nutrients and vitamins from diet alone. This is because food today, whether "organic" or otherwise, is treated with ridiculous amounts of chemicals. Supplements help redress the imbalance, and in some cases counteract the effects of modern life.

You may do well without any supplementation at all—but it's not optimal. And if you're reading this book, **you're clearly not interested in average.** The only way to determine whether you have a deficiency and you require a particular supplement is through a blood test. There are a few core supplements we'll cover in depth in this chapter. This list is by no means exhaustive, and entire books have been written on the subject, so I recommend you do further reading. But in the end, it's not about how many supplements you take. All that matters is how effective they are. Choosing to focus on a few and taking them regularly is likely to have more impact on your health, as opposed to having a cupboard full and taking them haphazardly.

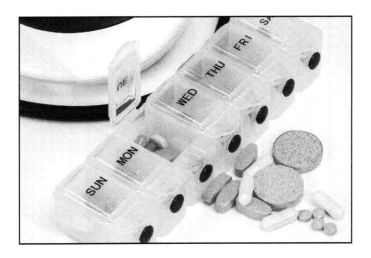

## OMEGA-3s

Omega-3s are essential fatty acids that play an important role in health, and they cannot be produced by the human body. The main omega-3 fatty acids are alpha-linolenic acid (ALA), docosahexaenoic acid (DHA), and eicosapentaenoic acid (EPA). ALA is found mainly in plant-based foods such as flaxseeds, chia seeds, and walnuts, whereas DHA and EPA are mainly found in fish.

The outstanding benefit of omega-3s is their anti-inflammatory and antioxidant effect. Chronic inflammation is the root cause of most disease. Therefore, the less inflammation you have, the better your chances of disease prevention. Omega-3s have been linked to improved cardiovascular function and reduced coronary events. Their potential to improve cognitive function in Alzheimer's patients is also promising.[155]

---

155    Daniel Kellyle Swanson, Robert Block, and Shaker A. Mousa, "Omega-3 Fatty Acids EPA and DHA: Health Benefits Throughout Life," *Advances in Nutrition*, Volume 3, Issue 1, 1 January 2012: 1–7, https://doi.org/10.3945/an.111.000893.

According to research, omega-3 deficiency is one of the top 10 causes of death in America.[156] This is because the typical Western diet has an omega-6 to omega-3 ratio of 20:1, whereas the ideal is 1:1! Too much omega-6 in your diet can result in chronic inflammation. Studies show omega-3s can improve sperm motility,[157] and infertile men tend to have lower levels of omega-3s. The bottom line? As a young man, both for disease prevention and optimal fertility, you need to supplement with omega-3s.

There are two main ways to get omega-3s in your diet. First is through eating fish (e.g., salmon, tuna, cod) at least a couple times a week. But given pollution in the environment and the disputable "freshness" of any fish, alone it's unlikely to net you enough omega-3s. Be aware that canned tuna does not count because it has been stripped of most of its omega-3s.

The other way to get omega-3s, and I recommend you do this regardless, is through supplementation. You can choose either fish oil capsules or cod liver oil. According to P.D. Mangan, author of *Best Supplements for Men's Health, Strength, and Virility*, capsules are not recommended due to the distribution process, which means they sit on shelves for months at a time. The oil then becomes oxidized, which negates the benefits and even becomes harmful. Mangan recommends cod liver oil because the bottles are tightly sealed and

---

156    Goodarz Danaei, Eric L. Ding, Dariush Mozaffarian, Ben Taylor, Jürgen Rehm, Christopher J. L. Murray and Majid Ezzati, "The Preventable Causes of Death in the United States: Comparative Risk Assessment of Dietary, Lifestyle, and Metabolic Risk Factors," *PLoS Med*, 2009 Apr, 6(4): e1000058, published online 2009 Apr 28, doi: 10.1371/journal.pmed.1000058.

157    Hosseini B, Nourmohamadi M, Hajipour S, Taghizadeh M, Asemi Z, Keshavarz SA, Jafarnejad S, "The Effect of Omega-3 Fatty Acids, EPA, and/or DHA on Male Infertility: A Systematic Review and Meta-analysis," *J Diet Suppl*, 2018 Feb 16: 1–12, doi: 10.1080/19390211.2018.1431753.

flushed with nitrogen to prevent oxidation.[158] I use cod liver oil for this reason and have had great success with it—just don't expect it to taste good!

RECOMMENDED DOSAGE: A minimum dosage of Omega-3s should be 1,000 mg a day. But as Dr. Brett Osborn states, "All fish oil is not created equal." You must be wary in choosing fish oils because most are laden with omega-6s, so check the label to see how much omega-3 you're actually getting. Dr. Osborn recommends you supplement aggressively with up to 3,000 mg a day.[159]

## MAGNESIUM

Magnesium is an essential macromineral responsible for a number of functions in the body. These include normal nerve function, muscle contraction and relaxation, heart rhythm, and bone mineral health. Magnesium works to create energy in your body in the form of adenosine triphosphate (ATP), as well as ensuring you have a good night's rest.

Low magnesium intake is linked to high blood pressure, stroke, calcification of soft tissue, and arterial plaque buildup. Magnesium deficiency also appears to play a role in insulin resistance, suggesting a link between deficiency and type 2 diabetes.[160] Magnesium is abundant in many foods; examples include oatmeal, almonds, spinach, and sunflower seeds. However, it's unlikely the food you eat will contain enough magnesium, and the average American diet is almost devoid of magnesium.

---

158   P.D. Mangan, *Best Supplements for Men's Health, Strength, and Virility: A Concise, Scientific Guide to Maintaining Youth, Vigor, and Manhood* (Phalanx Press, 2014).

159   Dr. Brett Osborn, *Get Serious: A Neurosurgeon's Guide to Optimal Health and Fitness* (Book Publishers Network, 2014).

160   Samantha Long and Andrea MP Romani, "Role of Cellular Magnesium in Human Diseases," *Austin J Nutr Food Sci*, 2014 Nov 18, 2(10): 1051, published online 2014 Nov 18.

Magnesium levels have been linked with testosterone levels. In a study of 399 men aged 65 years or older, there was a significant association with magnesium, total testosterone, and IGF-1.[161] Aim to supplement with magnesium tabs or oil on a daily basis. Personally, I prefer to use magnesium oil, as I believe it absorbs better through the skin. It's not actually an oil—it's a spray. The name originates from the oily texture when magnesium chloride flakes are mixed in with water.

I like to apply magnesium before going to bed, especially on muscles sore from training, as it promotes a relaxing effect. If you choose to use magnesium oil and you have sensitive skin, you may get a rash from using it. It's nothing to worry about, but it probably means you can't use the spray and you should use tablets instead.

RECOMMENDED DOSAGE: Magnesium should be a mainstay in your supplement stack, particularly if you want a restful night's sleep. With the spray, it's not very scientific; I just tend to spray a couple of times on my skin. You should experiment with this dosage and judge how you feel on it. If you feel sleepy or sedate on this dose, look to lower the dose accordingly.

It appears adequate magnesium concentrations can also influence the affinity of testosterone to SHBG, resulting in more free testosterone.[162] Dr. Rob Kominiarek recommends all men undergoing TRT supplement with 400 mg of magnesium glycinate daily, as

---

161    Maggio M, Ceda GP, Lauretani F, Cattabiani C, Avantaggiato E, Morganti S, Ablondi F, Bandinelli S, Dominguez LJ, Barbagallo M, Paolisso G, Semba RD, Ferrucci L, "Magnesium and anabolic hormones in older men," *Int J Androl*, 2011 Dec, 34(6 Pt 2): e594–600, doi: 10.1111/j.1365-2605.2011.01193.x.

162    Marcello Maggio, Francesca De Vita, Fulvio Lauretani, Antonio Nouvenne, Tiziana Meschi, Andrea Ticinesi, Ligia J. Dominguez, Mario Barbagallo, Elisabetta Dall'Aglio, and Gian Paolo Ceda, "The Interplay between Magnesium and Testosterone in Modulating Physical Function in Men," *Int J Endocrinol*, 2014: 525249, published online 2014 Mar 3, doi: 10.1155/2014/525249.

testosterone can deplete intracellular magnesium due to its effects on neurotransmitter pathways. You should also take magnesium if you work out, as strenuous exercise may increase magnesium requirements by 10–20%.[163]

## VITAMIN D

Despite its name, vitamin D is actually a pro-hormone and not a vitamin. It is a vital nutrient for human health and contributes to bone growth and hormone synthesis, among other things.

There are two forms of vitamin D: D2 and D3. Vitamin D2 is found mostly in plant-based foods such as mushrooms. Vitamin D3 can be found in small quantities in foods such as eggs and fish. The one to supplement with is vitamin D3, as this is more effective in comparison to D2. Vitamin D is a fat-soluble nutrient, meaning it is absorbed through fat. Therefore, you should take vitamin D3 with a meal. I use a cod liver oil supplement fortified with vitamin D3, and the fatty acids in the fish oil aid absorption.

After several weeks of supplementing this way, I went from vitamin D deficiency to optimal levels, as confirmed by a blood test. Although you can get vitamin D through food and supplements, it's thought 80–90% of it is synthesized when the body is exposed to sunlight.

We've all been told about the importance of protecting our skin from the sun, but covering up from the sun could actually prevent us from getting enough vitamin D. It appears sunscreen with SPF of 30 or more can reduce vitamin D synthesis by up to 95% because of reduced exposure to the sun.[164] However, if your skin is sensitive

163    Nielsen FH, Lukaski HC, "Update on the relationship between magnesium and exercise," *Magnes Res*, 2006 Sep, 19(3): 180–9.

164    Matsuoka LY, Ide L, Wortsman J, MacLaughlin JA, Holick MF, "Sunscreens suppress cutaneous vitamin D3 synthesis," *J Clin Endocrinol Metab*, 1987 Jun, 64(6): 1165–8.

to the sun (as in my case), you may have no choice but to use a high factor sunscreen. That's why it's even more important to supplement with vitamin D.

Vitamin D deficiency affects almost 50% of the population worldwide and is associated with increased mortality, cancer, cardiovascular disease, depression, bone fractures, diabetes, and autoimmune disease.[165] Given we spend most of our time indoors, and if you live in a climate with limited sunshine, vitamin D supplementation suddenly becomes critical.

RECOMMENDED DOSAGE: You should supplement aggressively with vitamin D. But don't overdo it; too much can lead to calcium toxicity, although you'd have to take a lot for that to happen. Nevertheless, that's why it is crucial to buy a vitamin D supplement containing vitamin K2. These vitamins work in synergy together, and the presence of vitamin K2 helps counteract the negative effects of high-dose vitamin D3.[166]

The best way to determine if you have vitamin D deficiency (and chances are you do) is through a blood test, and you should aim to reach a level of 50–65 ng/ml (125–162.5 nmol/L). Depending on the outcome of your blood test, you should aim to take between 1,000–10,000 IU daily.[167] If you have a low level of vitamin D, it may be a good idea to supplement aggressively. In my experience however, most people do well with 3000-5000 IU daily.

---

165    Rathish Nair and Arun Maseeh, "Vitamin D: The 'sunshine' vitamin," *J Pharmacol Pharmacother*, 2012 Apr–Jun, 3(2): 118–126, doi: 10.4103/0976-500X.95506.

166    Adriana J. van Ballegooijen, Stefan Pilz, Andreas Tomaschitz, Martin R. Grübler, and Nicolas Verheyen, "The Synergistic Interplay between Vitamins D and K for Bone and Cardiovascular Health: A Narrative Review," *Int J Endocrinol*, 2017: 7454376, published online 2017 Sep 12, doi: 10.1155/2017/7454376.

167    Osborn, *Get Serious.*

## VITAMIN B COMPLEX

A vitamin B complex is usually made up of the following B vitamins: B1 (thiamine), B2 (riboflavin), B3 (niacin), B5 (pantothenic acid), B6 (pyridoxine), B7 (biotin), B9 (folic acid) and B12 (cobalamin). Vitamin B can also be found in meat, dairy, and leafy greens.

B complex is important for a process called methylation. This process is vital to DNA repair, cognition, and immune function among others. Suboptimal vitamin B12 levels are associated with increased cardiovascular risk, and low vitamin B appears to be associated with increased cancer risk, due to its role in the DNA repair process.[168] Indeed, impaired methylation is linked to elevated homocysteine levels, a risk factor for cardiovascular disease, and high folate (vitamin B12) intake reduces homocysteine levels.[169]

In studies on the effect of multivitamins on health markers, it appears the presence of high levels of vitamin B are the deciding factor. Vitamin B supplementation has also been shown to improve mood. Indeed, multiple studies associate multivitamin supplementation with reduced cardiovascular risk. And once more, although wholly conclusive, it seems high levels of vitamin B are a contributing factor.[170]

RECOMMENDED DOSAGE: Dr. Brett Osborn recommends taking a B complex that has the most folic acid per tablet—up to 400

---

168    Milly Ryan-Harshman, PhD RD, Walid Aldoori, MB BCh MPA ScD, "Vitamin B12 and health," *Can Fam Physician*, 2008 Apr, 54(4): 536–541.

169    David A Bender, "Daily doses of multivitamin tablets. Regular consumption will probably do you no good, with a few exceptions," *BMJ*, 2002 Jul 27, 325(7357): 173–174.

170    David O. Kennedy, "B Vitamins and the Brain: Mechanisms, Dose and Efficacy—A Review," *Nutrients*, 2016 Feb; 8(2): 68, published online 2016 Jan 28, doi: 10.3390/nu8020068.

mcg of folic acid, to be precise.[171] As there are multiple vitamins in a B complex supplement, the exact dosage can vary by manufacturer. The reference daily intake (RDI) for the individual nutrients are as follows:

- B1 (thiamine) 1.2 mg
- B2 (riboflavin) 1.3 mg
- B3 (niacin) 16 mg
- B5 (pantothenic acid) 5 mg—suggested amount, as there is no RDI available
- B6 (pyridoxine) 1.3 mg
- B7 (biotin) 30 mcg—suggested amount, as there is no RDI available
- B9 (folate) 400 mcg
- B12 (cobalamin) 2.4 mg

Aim to find a B-complex that has a micronutrient profile as close to the above as possible. Take one tablet a day.

## MULTIVITAMIN

Nowadays, it's pretty tough to get a balanced intake through food alone. This is because today's food has NO RESEMBLANCE to the food your grandparents ate. It's sprayed with pesticides and who knows what else. But not only that, it remains on shelves for weeks. So it's any wonder most food is lacking in vital nutrients. In light of this, I would say taking a multivitamin is a necessity to ensure you get an adequate intake of proper nutrients.

Two double-blind placebo studies looked at bodyweight and composition differences in obese individuals for 15 weeks. The groups were divided into two; one group took a placebo, while the other took a multivitamin and mineral supplement. The researchers found men

---

171  Osborn, *Get Serious.*

in the multivitamin supplement group had lower body weight, less fat mass, and more energy expenditure.[172] It also appears a multivitamin can play a role in disease prevention, for example by lowering the risk of cancer. Because, ultimately, it's chronic nutrient shortfalls that lead to disease.[173]

RECOMMENDED DOSAGE: I can't give a standard dosage recommendation for multivitamins because it really depends on the strength of each macronutrient in it. Therefore, you're best off following the advice of the manufacturer here. If you can find a multivitamin that combines some of the supplements above in sufficient dosages, such as vitamin D or B12, then get it by all means. Although, it's unlikely a multivitamin will have individual micronutrients in the quantities you require to be in optimal health.

According to Dr. Brett Osborn, you should steer clear of single tablet preparation multivitamins. This is because the dosage of micronutrients will be quite low, whereas multi-tablet preps contain higher quantities. In addition, taking multi-tablets (e.g., nine tablets of Life Extension® Mix), means you will have a steady supply of micronutrients around the clock, which is far better for your health.

---

172   Major GC, Doucet E, Jacqmain M, St-Onge M, Bouchard C, Tremblay A, "Multivitamin and dietary supplements, body weight and appetite: results from a cross-sectional and a randomised double-blind placebo-controlled study," *Br J Nutr*, 2008 May, 99(5): 1157–67. Epub 2007 Nov 1.

173   Elizabeth Ward, "Addressing nutritional gaps with multivitamin and mineral supplements," *Nutr J*, 2014, 13: 72, published online 2014 Jul 15, doi: 10.1186/1475-2891-13-72.

# CHAPTER 9

# THE TESTOSTERONE MYTH

Testosterone is still widely demonized despite the positive effects it has on male health. And despite the fact credible information on the subject exists in the form of clinical studies and research, misinformation still abounds. At this stage, maybe you think you have low testosterone, but you're reluctant to undergo a medication for fear of the side effects. That's terribly unfortunate—testosterone is crucial to male health. If that's the case, why is there so much stigma around testosterone?

We've long been told high levels of testosterone in men cause a string of negative characteristics. Apparently, men with elevated testosterone levels are dangerous, impulsive, reckless, and have an insatiable sexual appetite. What's more, therapeutic testosterone is taken with a physician's prescription and is completely LEGAL. And yet, it's still often viewed as something nefarious and black market.

Despite the information available at our fingertips, thanks to the Internet, many still buy into the countless myths about testosterone. And if you tell a lie for long enough, it eventually becomes accepted as fact. But the lies end here and now. In this chapter I will RIP APART the myths on testosterone and put the bullshit to bed once and for all.

## MYTH #1: TESTOSTERONE CAUSES AGGRESSION

One of the most common myths about testosterone is that high concentrations provoke aggressive and violent behavior. Men ask me all the time, "Does testosterone make you angry?" Popular culture portrays men with high testosterone levels as mindless, thuggish brutes. Yet, several studies showed exogenous testosterone administration did not result in aggressive behavior and mood swings in healthy men. In one study, a group of men were given either 200 mg of testosterone enanthate, or 200 mg sodium chloride biweekly for eight weeks. No significant responses were noted in the control group. However, *significant* reductions in negative mood (tension, anger, and fatigue) were noted in the group that was administered testosterone.[174]

One landmark study was undertaken in 1996 on 40 men to monitor the effect of supraphysiologic doses of testosterone on muscle size and strength. The men received either 600 mg of testosterone enanthate or a placebo via intramuscular injection weekly for 10 weeks. Using a Multidimensional Anger Inventory assessment (i.e., a questionnaire to measure subjective feelings of anger), researchers found **no significant differences** between the testosterone and control groups. Not only that, but no significant changes in mood or behavior were reported by the men *or* their live-in partners during the study.[175]

In a placebo-controlled study, 56 men age 20–50 were administered up to 600 mg of testosterone cypionate per week, separated by six weeks without treatment. Minimal psychiatric effects were observed in 84% of the subjects, 12% became mildly hypomanic, and 4% markedly hypomanic. The researchers concluded 300 mg a week of testosterone (more than a clinical dose) produces few psychiatric

---

174    O'Connor DB, Archer J, Hair WM, Wu FC, "Exogenous testosterone, aggression, and mood in eugonadal and hypogonadal men," *Physiol Behav*, 2002 Apr 1, 75(4): 557–66.

175    Bhasin S, Storer TW, Berman N, Callegari C, Clevenger B, Phillips J, Bunnell TJ, Tricker R, Shirazi A, Casaburi R, "The effects of supraphysiologic doses of testosterone on muscle size and strength in normal men," *N Engl J Med*, 1996 Jul 4, 335(1): 1–7.

effects, whereas doses of 500 mg or more per week may produce occasional "prominent manic or hypomanic reactions."[176]

A further study investigated the link between exogenous testosterone and aggressive behavior in dominant and impulsive men. They found testosterone on its own **did not increase aggressive behavior**. But testosterone appeared to increase aggressive behavior in men who scored high in trait dominance or low in trait self-control.[177] This confirms my own observation and those of other men on TRT: Testosterone doesn't change your personality. If anything, it accentuates your existing traits.

Even at high (supraphysiologic) doses, testosterone does not cause you to rampage through the streets in an orgy of violence like Wesley Snipes from *Demolition Man*. So if men don't experience adverse reactions from taking 600 mg a week of testosterone, it's **not going to happen** on a therapeutic dose of 200 mg a week.

There is a broad spectrum of what actually constitutes aggressive behavior—from aggressiveness to physical violence.[178] Yet, there is a marked difference between impulsive, unrestrained violence and the channeled, calm aggression men experience with optimized testosterone levels. Training intensely in the gym and using aggression positively to attack weights doesn't mean you'll go out and attack people. It doesn't work like that.

---

176   Bhasin S, Woodhouse L, Casaburi R, Singh AB, Bhasin D, Berman N, Chen X, Yarasheski KE, Magliano L, Dzekov C, Dzekov J, Bross R, Phillips J, Sinha-Hikim I, Shen R, Storer TW, "Testosterone dose-response relationships in healthy young men," *Am J Physiol Endocrinol Metab*, 2001 Dec, 281(6): E1172–81.

177   Carré JM, Geniole SN, Ortiz TL, Bird BM, Videto A, Bonin PL, "Exogenous Testosterone Rapidly Increases Aggressive Behavior in Dominant and Impulsive Men," *Biol Psychiatry*, (Aug 2017) 82(4): 249–256.

178   Menelaos L. Batrinos, "Testosterone and Aggressive Behavior in Man," *Int J Endocrinol Metab*, 2012 Summer, 10(3): 563–568, published online 2012 Jun 30, doi: 10.5812/ijem.3661.

But anyone with two brain cells can see most men can control their urges. And the men who form the basis for the link between testosterone and aggression are often: a) already unhinged, and/or b) abusing testosterone. These individuals are often predisposed to recreational drugs and alcohol abuse. And so this mix of anabolics and drugs creates a lethal cocktail resulting in manic behavior.

Researchers hypothesize a high testosterone-cortisol ratio may actually be responsible for socially aggressive behavior.[179] In his excellent book *American Biohacker*, Russ Scala, founder of Scala Precision Health, states the testosterone-cortisol ratio is of prime importance.[180] And according to Scala, mood swings and aggressive behavior can result from imbalance between estrogen, serotonin, dopamine, and testosterone—not just testosterone itself. So when this delicate balance is disrupted, aggressive or manic depressive episodes manifest. Indeed, first responders such as military veterans and law enforcement can become vulnerable to testosterone-cortisol imbalance due to the chronic stress of their professions.

## MYTH #2: TESTOSTERONE CAUSES PROSTATE CANCER

Perhaps one of the biggest myths about testosterone is that it causes prostate cancer. Few realize that the correlation between testosterone and prostate cancer is based on a **single study from 1941 that involved two men.**[181] The two men in the study both had low

179   Mehta PH, Josephs RA, "Testosterone and cortisol jointly regulate dominance: evidence for a dual-hormone hypothesis," *Horm Behav*, 2010 Nov, 58(5): 898–906, doi: 10.1016/j.yhbeh.2010.08.020.

180   Russ Scala, *American Biohacker: Saving Lives Since 1975* (Archangel Ink, 2017).

181   Charles Huggins and Clarence V. Hodges, "Studies on Prostatic Cancer. I. The Effect of Castration, of Estrogen and of Androgen Injection on Serum Phosphatases in Metastatic Carcinoma of the Prostate," American Associates for Cancer Research, DOI: Published April 1941.

testosterone, and one developed prostate cancer after being administered testosterone. To be clear, this IS NOT definitive science. Yet the medical community still buys into the idea that testosterone promotes prostate cancer. It's complete lunacy. Study after study has shown there is **no link between prostate cancer and testosterone**, and several studies actually associate <u>chronic low testosterone</u> with increased prostate cancer risk.[182]

One large-scale study investigated the link between androgens (i.e., male sex hormones) and prostate cancer in men. The participants were divided into two groups—those treated with dutasteride (a drug used to treat enlarged prostate) and those given a placebo.

The study is significant because it involved a large number of participants—8,122 men in total, and of those, 3,242 men who had at least one prior negative prostate biopsy (i.e., all clear for prostate cancer) received a placebo. The men had prostate exams at two- and four-year intervals to detect any prostate irregularities. In the placebo group, the researchers found **no association** between testosterone or DHT levels with prostate cancer.[183] Another study looking at the incidence of prostate cancer among men on TRT who had preexisting prostate conditions and were high-risk candidates for prostate cancer found no clear link between testosterone and prostate cancer.[184]

Finally, one meta-analysis looked at 19 different studies where hypogonadal (low testosterone) men received testosterone. All studies

182   Jason E. Michaud, Kevin L. Billups, and Alan W. Partin, "Testosterone and prostate cancer: an evidence-based review of pathogenesis and oncologic risk," *Ther Adv Urol*, 2015 Dec, 7(6): 378–387, doi: 10.1177/1756287215597633.

183   Jason E. Michaud, Kevin L. Billups, and Alan W. Partin, "Testosterone and prostate cancer: an evidence-based review of pathogenesis and oncologic risk," *Ther Adv Urol*, 2015 Dec, 7(6): 378–387, doi: 10.1177/1756287215597633.

184   Ranjith Ramasamy, Erik S. Fisher, and Peter N. Schlegel, "Testosterone replacement and prostate cancer," *Indian J Urol*, 2012 Apr–Jun, 28(2): 123–128, doi: 10.4103/0970-1591.98449.

were double-blind, randomized, placebo controlled only trials involving men age 45 years or older. This analysis involved 643 men receiving testosterone, and 427 receiving a placebo. The analysis concluded there was **no significant difference** in prostate cancer incidence between men on testosterone and a placebo.[185]

## MYTH #3: TESTOSTERONE CAUSES BALDNESS

Another classic myth is that testosterone causes baldness. It's funny; of all the perceived side effects of taking testosterone, the one that scares men most is the idea of losing their hair. This is primarily because they feel if they lose it, women will no longer find them attractive. But, in reality, a woman is more attracted to your confidence (the antithesis of low testosterone) and the way you carry yourself—NOT by how much hair you have.

The good news is that testosterone is **not directly responsible** for baldness. Androgenic alopecia or baldness is primarily a result of genetic and hormonal factors. Keeping or losing your hair is largely out of your control and is not determined by testosterone. One German study of 373 men examined the relationship between testosterone and male pattern baldness. Each participant had blood drawn to verify concentrations of sex hormones, and they abstained from prescription drugs in the seven days prior to the study. Dermatologists then checked participants to determine if they had hair loss or not (yes or no). The researchers concluded there was no observable link between sex hormone concentrations and male pattern baldness.[186]

---

185   Ranjith Ramasamy, Erik S. Fisher, and Peter N. Schlegel, "Testosterone replacement and prostate cancer," *Indian J Urol*, 2012 Apr–Jun, 28(2): 123–128, doi: 10.4103/0970-1591.98449.

186   Hanna Kische; Andreas Arnold; Stefan Gross; et al., "Sex Hormones and Hair Loss in Men From the General Population of Northeastern Germany," *JAMA Dermatol*, 2017, 153(9): 935–937, doi:10.1001/jamadermatol.2017.0297.

In the presence of elevated testosterone, dihydrotestosterone (DHT) levels increase through the conversion of testosterone via the 5-alpha reductase enzyme.[187] It's thought the main cause of hair loss in men is from elevated DHT levels because the presence of DHT stimulates androgen action on the scalp, decreasing hair follicle size and increasing the prevalence of shorter, finer hairs.[188] In other words, testosterone may accelerate hair loss IF you are already genetically predisposed to it.

At the time of writing, I have been on testosterone for three years and **haven't suffered any hair loss**. I consider myself fortunate because I'm not predisposed to hair loss. But even if testosterone accelerated hair loss, it wouldn't stop me from taking it. My life has been impacted so much by testosterone, that any "negative" from hair loss is more than made up for by increased libido, confidence, lean muscle, and overall well-being.

## MYTH #4: TESTOSTERONE TURNS YOU INTO A SEX ADDICT

Many are under the impression that elevating testosterone levels turns you into a sex-crazed maniac, and I think the reason why is because people today are testosterone deficient. Therefore, to them, a healthy interest in sex is seen as abnormal, as they have no sexual desire themselves!

---

187   Kishore M. Lakshman, Beth Kaplan, Thomas G. Travison, Shehzad Basaria, Philip E. Knapp, Atam B. Singh, Michael P. LaValley, Norman A. Mazer,a and Shalender Bhasina, "The Effects of Injected Testosterone Dose and Age on the Conversion of Testosterone to Estradiol and Dihydrotestosterone in Young and Older Men," *J Clin Endocrinol Metab*, 2010 Aug, 95(8): 3955–3964, published online 2010 Jun 9, doi: 10.1210/jc.2010-0102.

188   Lacey Hizartzidis, PhD, "Is There a Link Between Hair Loss and Testosterone Levels?" Medical News Bulletin, June 7, 2017, https://www.medicalnewsbulletin.com/link-hair-loss-testosterone-levels/.

A strong libido, a desire to have regular sex, is a NORMAL part of being a man. Evolution designed us to spread our seed. Would these moral puritans say 18-year-olds are immoral for constantly thinking about sex? Of course not, they'd say, "It's just their age!" So why the hell is it wrong for a grown man taking testosterone to have a strong libido? Suddenly, he's a sex maniac? Please ...

Our society is a kind of paradox. On the one hand, popular culture—especially the film and music industries—sexualizes virtually everything. But on the other hand, being a man and having a sex drive is somehow wrong or immoral. If the puritanical zealots had their way, you'd remain a sexless virgin. The thing to understand is that anecdotal stories of men with a crazy sex drive from testosterone usually involve massive doses of testosterone, which has nothing to do with safe therapeutic doses of testosterone.

One study of healthy male volunteers age 60–75 years old examined the effect of dose-dependent testosterone on sexual function, mood, and cognition. Participants were given intramuscular testosterone enanthate injections per week of 25, 50, 125, 300, or 600 mg for 20 weeks. The researchers concluded that free testosterone levels were positively correlated with improved sexual function, morning erections, spontaneous erections, and libido. Interestingly, they found intercourse and masturbation frequency <u>did not increase</u>,[189] suggesting even at supraphysiologic doses of 600 mg a week, testosterone does not turn you into a sex addict.

---

189     Peter B. Gray, Atam B. Singh, Linda J. Woodhouse, Thomas W. Storer, Richard Casaburi, Jeanne Dzekov, Connie Dzekov, Indrani Sinha-Hikim, Shalender Bhasin, "Dose-Dependent Effects of Testosterone on Sexual Function, Mood, and Visuospatial Cognition in Older Men," *The Journal of Clinical Endocrinology & Metabolism*, Volume 90, Issue 7, 1 July 2005: 3838–3846, https://doi.org/10.1210/jc.2005-0247.

# MYTH #5: LOW TESTOSTERONE IS PART OF GROWING OLD

One idea that has gained popularity recently is that taking testosterone goes against nature. In this cozy, gumdrop fantasyland, we all age gracefully and die of natural causes. But the proponents of this idea fail to recognize that nature never intended us to become frail, weak, and completely useless as we grow old. We live in an UNNATURAL environment full of chemicals and toxins. Therefore, to live as nature intended, in certain instances we may have to resort to UNNATURAL measures to live a life of vitality. Should we just lie down and accept average health, because it goes against someone's sensibilities of what constitutes "natural"?

In fact, research suggests an age-related decline in testosterone is not necessarily natural at all. This was demonstrated in an Australian study spanning five years that measured testosterone changes in 1,588 men age 35 or older. The researchers concluded, "an age related decline in T levels is **not inevitable,**" but is largely due to lifestyle factors.[190] Therefore, having low testosterone as we grow older is NOT something we should accept. Have you ever seen those pictures taken by intrepid explorers who encountered isolated tribes in Papua New Guinea and the Amazon rainforest? The old men were all ripped to shreds and giving the 1,000-yard stare. It sure as hell didn't look like low testosterone was an inevitable result of growing old in their society.

The irony is that if these people who are against testosterone developed cancer or diabetes, they would not hesitate to seek treatment for it. Does that go against nature? The fact is, nature

---

190    Zumin Shi Andre B. Araujo Sean Martin Peter O'Loughlin Gary A. Wittert, "Longitudinal Changes in Testosterone Over Five Years in Community-Dwelling Men," *The Journal of Clinical Endocrinology & Metabolism*, Volume 98, Issue 8, 1 August 2013: 3289–3297, https://doi.org/10.1210/jc.2012-3842.

never planned for human beings to be so out of touch with their environment and to live in a toxic cesspit. Therefore, **hormone optimization is simply restoring your health** to what nature *intended* before this chemical onslaught.

In this chapter, we've debunked many of the common myths surrounding testosterone. However, scientific research aside—think about it logically for a moment. How on EARTH can a *hormone* that your body produces naturally be in any way bad for you? Especially when taken in doses that mimic the body's own natural production. By now you should understand that, far from being a negative force, testosterone is a force for good in your life and in the world. And in the next chapter, we're going to look at just how beneficial testosterone is for your health.

# CHAPTER 10

# THE POWER OF TESTOSTERONE

Today, the mainstream consensus is that too much testosterone is bad for you. In fact, there are many in society who feel testosterone is evil and is the source of everything that's wrong in the world. Yet the reality is that low testosterone is a destructive force, particularly on male health. Testosterone is not only a force for good, but is fundamental to every man's health and well-being.

In this chapter, we'll take a deep dive into how testosterone benefits your health. The majority of the literature focuses on the effects of testosterone replacement therapy. Nevertheless, testosterone is testosterone, so when you optimize your testosterone levels, you'll see benefits to your health whether you undergo TRT or optimize your testosterone naturally. And if you do undergo TRT, this chapter is proof positive of how safe it really is. Among other things, we'll look at how testosterone improves symptoms of depression, increases muscle mass, and improves your sex life.

## TESTOSTERONE AND DEPRESSION

We've all struggled with some form of depression at one time or another; it's a debilitating condition that leaves you feeling helpless. Yet, despite our creature comforts and immense abundance, we still struggle with it, and the high rate of depression we see in society today is actually a modern phenomenon. Indeed, studies show depression rates differ significantly between modernized, rural, and traditional communities.[191]

---

191 Brandon H Hidaka, "Depression as a disease of modernity: explanations for increasing prevalence," *J Affect Disord*, 2012 Nov, 140(3): 205–214.

Depression can be caused by a number of things, including bio-chemical imbalance, genetics, and stressful life events.[192] In order to combat depression, physicians often prescribe antidepressants (SSRIs), and counseling with a therapist is often recommended. While these methods may alleviate some symptoms of depression, oftentimes they do not address the root cause of the depression.

An underlying cause commonly overlooked by both studies and physicians alike is hormonal imbalance—particularly low testos-terone. Low testosterone is strongly linked to depression, anxiety, and lack of motivation.[193] Studies show a correlation between low testosterone levels and incidence of depression.[194] One particular study investigated depressive symptoms in 200 men with serum tes-tosterone levels between 200 and 350 ng/dL (6.9–12 nmol/L). The researchers found symptoms were present in 56% of subjects more than twice the rate of the general population,[195] demonstrating a clear correlation between low testosterone and depressive states. And additional research shows testosterone to have an antidepressant and

192   Bondy Brigitta, MD, "Pathophysiology of depression and mechanisms of treatment," *Dialogues Clin Neurosci*, 2002 Mar, 4(1): 7–20.

193   Mario Amore, Marco Innamorati, Sara Costi, Leo Sher, Paolo Girardi, Maurizio Pompili, "Partial Androgen Deficiency, Depression, and Testosterone Supplementation in Aging Men," *Int J Endocrinol*, 2012: 280724, published online 2012 Jun 7, doi: 10.1155/2012/280724.

194   Shores MM1, Moceri VM, Sloan KL, Matsumoto AM, Kivlahan DR, "Low testosterone levels predict incident depressive illness in older men: effects of age and medical morbidity," *J Clin Psychiatry*, 2005 Jan, 66(1): 7–14.

195   Westley CJ, Amdur RL, Irwig MS, "High Rates of Depression and Depressive Symptoms among Men Referred for Borderline Testosterone Levels," *J Sex Med*, 2015 Aug, 12(8): 1753–60, doi: 10.1111/jsm.12937. Epub 2015 Jun 30.

anxiolytic (i.e., anxiety-reducing) effect.[196,197] Testosterone supplementation was shown to increase positive mood parameters in men with low testosterone, including friendliness, energy, and sense of well-being, and decreased negative mood parameters such as anger and irritability.[198]

## TESTOSTERONE AND MUSCLE MASS

One of the headline benefits of testosterone is the ability to increase strength and muscle mass. Sadly, our society sees weakness as a virtue, and a result, many men think muscles are for bodybuilders and gym rats only. However, building muscle is about more than looking good.

Aside from the mental benefits of feeling more confident, muscle improves insulin sensitivity and is crucial in controlling blood glucose levels, protecting against diseases such as diabetes.[199] Muscle improves metabolic rate, meaning the more you have, the more calories you burn at rest. So, essentially, gaining muscle turns you into a fat-burning machine!

In addition, muscle acts as a storage depot for protein, and in disease states such as cancer, sepsis (a toxic response to infection), or traumatic injury, amino acid proteins are released from muscle

196   Peter Celec, Daniel Kellya Ostatníková, and Július Hodosy, "On the effects of testosterone on brain behavioral functions," *Front Neurosci*, 2015, 9: 12, published online 2015 Feb 17, doi: 10.3389/fnins.2015.00012.

197   Zarrouf FA, Artz S, Griffith J, Sirbu C, Kommor M, "Testosterone and depression: systematic review and meta-analysis," *J Psychiatr Pract*, 2009 Jul, 15(4): 289–305, doi: 10.1097/01.pra.0000358315.88931.fc.

198   Wang. C et al., "Testosterone replacement therapy improves mood in hypogonadal men—a clinical research center study," *J Clin Endocrinol Metab*, 1996 Oct, 81(10): 3578–83.

199   Alexandra C. McPherron, Tingqing Guo, Nichole D. Bond, Oksana Gavrilova, "Increasing muscle mass to improve metabolism," *Adipocyte*, 2013 Apr 1, 2(2): 92–98, published online 2013 Apr 1, doi: 10.4161/adip.22500.

tissue for wound healing.[200] This is why survival rates for cancer and traumatic injuries are much greater in those with high lean body mass. In fact, muscular strength is significantly associated with lower risk of death from all causes in men.[201] Ultimately, muscle is vital to everyday life from picking up objects, to deterring would-be attackers, to attracting a mate.

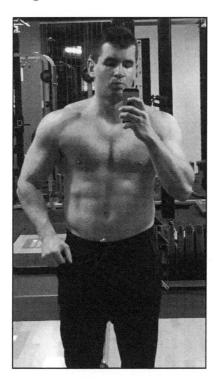

Low testosterone is associated with reduced muscle mass, which is likely due to reduced muscle protein synthesis.[202] I've experienced

200    Osborn, Get Serious.

201    Jonatan R Ruiz, Xuemei Sui, Felipe Lobelo, James R Morrow, Jr, Allen W Jackson, Michael Sjöström, Steven N Blair, "Association between muscular strength and mortality in men: prospective cohort study," BMJ, 2008 Jul 12, 337(7661): 92–95, doi: 10.1136/bmj.a439.

202    Cobo G et al., "Hypogonadism associated with muscle atrophy, physical inactivity and ESA hyporesponsiveness in men undergoing haemodialysis," Nefrologia, 2017 Jan–Feb, 37(1): 54–60, doi: 10.1016/j.nefro.2016.04.009. Epub 2016 Aug 21.

this firsthand where I found it extremely difficult, if not impossible, to gain muscle with low testosterone. Testosterone improves strength and muscle mass primarily through increasing muscle protein synthesis.[203,204,205] However, it's not clear from the literature whether its action on muscle protein synthesis is direct or indirect. In one Australian study of 13 healthy, non-athletic, men age 21–37, 200 mg of intramuscular testosterone enanthate injection resulted in a 9.6% increase in fat-free mass, a bodyweight increase of 5%, and muscle strength increase of up to 19.2%.[206]

In another study, where exercise and nutritional intake were closely controlled, seven hypogonadal men age 19–47 were given 100 mg of testosterone enanthate a week for 10 weeks. The researchers noted increases in body weight, fat-free mass, and significant improvements in muscle strength.[207] And in one double-blind placebo study, 101 subjects with cirrhosis (liver disease) and low serum testosterone were given testosterone undecanoate (Nebido/Aveed) for 12 months. Their body composition was measured at 6 and 12 months. The

---

203   Brodsky IG, Balagopal P, Nair KS, "Effects of testosterone replacement on muscle mass and muscle protein synthesis in hypogonadal men—a clinical research center study," *J Clin Endocrinol Metab*, 1996 Oct, 81(10): 3469–75.

204   Griggs RC1, Kingston W, Jozefowicz RF, Herr BE, Forbes G, Halliday D, "Effect of testosterone on muscle mass and muscle protein synthesis," *J Appl Physiol* (1985), 1989 Jan, 66(1): 498–503.

205   Herbst KL, Bhasin S, "Testosterone action on skeletal muscle," *Curr Opin Clin Nutr Metab Care*, 2004 May, 7(3): 271–7.

206   Young NR, Baker HW, Liu G, Seeman E, "Body composition and muscle strength in healthy men receiving testosterone enanthate for contraception," *J Clin Endocrinol Metab*, 1993 Oct, 77(4): 1028–32.

207   Shalender Bhasin et al., "Testosterone Replacement Increases Fat-Free Mass and Muscle Size in Hypogonadal Men," *The Journal of Clinical Endocrinology & Metabolism*, Volume 82, Issue 2, 1 February 1997: 407–413, https://doi.org/10.1210/jcem.82.2.3733.

subjects treated with testosterone showed increases in fat-free mass and increased muscle mass.[208]

## TESTOSTERONE AND SEX

Physical intimacy is an essential part of being a man, and evolution designed us to spread our seed. Our desire to procreate is so strong that if you don't fulfill this basic biological need, life becomes very unpleasant. And central to your sexual well-being as a man is testosterone. Studies show testosterone improves feelings of sexual desire and arousal.[209] Testosterone is also crucial to maintaining proper penile function and erectile strength. Exogenous testosterone is often indicated in men with hypogonadism who suffer from erectile dysfunction (ED). One meta-analysis looked at the association between testosterone and erectile dysfunction in studies ranging from 1966–1998. They found the average positive response to treatment for erectile dysfunction was 16.7% with a placebo, and 65.4% in the groups treated with testosterone.[210,211] In other words, testosterone has a profound impact on both the mental and physical aspects of sex.

In another study, 31 men age 21–40 years old were given 200 mg of testosterone enanthate supplementation for four weeks. The purpose

---

208    Sinclair M, Grossmann M, Hoermann R, Angus PW, Gow PJ, "Testosterone therapy increases muscle mass in men with cirrhosis and low testosterone: A randomised controlled trial," *J Hepatol*, 2016 Nov, 65(5): 906–913, doi: 10.1016/j.jhep.2016.06.007.

209    Corona G, Isidori AM, Aversa A, Burnett AL, Maggi M, "Endocrinologic Control of Men's Sexual Desire and Arousal/Erection," *J Sex Med*, 2016 Mar, 13(3): 317–37, doi: 10.1016/j.jsxm.2016.01.007.

210    Jacob Rajfer, MD, "Relationship Between Testosterone and Erectile Dysfunction," *Rev Urol*, 2000 Spring, 2(2): 122–128.

211    Farid Saad et al., "Effects of testosterone on erectile function: implications for the therapy of erectile dysfunction," *BJU INTERNATIONAL*, 2007, 99, 988–992, doi:10.1111/j.1464-410X.2007.06756.x.

was to monitor the effect of testosterone on sexual mood and behavior. The groups were split into those receiving a placebo versus testosterone. The testosterone group showed significant interest in sex compared to the placebo group. Interestingly however, the authors noted that testosterone did not increase frequency of sexual intercourse, masturbation, or erections.[212]

A separate study spanning 1987–2004 examined the relationship between libido and testosterone levels in aging men. It evaluated 1632 men age 40–70 years who completed questionnaires on self-reported feelings and thoughts of sexual desire. The researchers also evaluated the total and free testosterone levels of these men, and they found a significant correlation between libido and testosterone concentrations.[213]

## TESTOSTERONE AND COGNITION

*The Oxford Dictionary* defines *cognition* as, "the mental action or process of acquiring knowledge and understanding through thought, experience, and the senses."[214] This process includes memory, decision-making, judgment, and evaluation. And the acquisition of knowledge, proper judgment, and decision-making fundamental to your success as a man.

Studies show low testosterone is associated with diminished cognition, while optimal levels of testosterone improve aspects of

---

212   Anderson RA, Bancroft J, Wu FC, "The effects of exogenous testosterone on sexuality and mood of normal men," *J Clin Endocrinol Metab*, 1992 Dec, 75(6): 1503–7.

213   Thomas G. Travison, John E. Morley, Andre B. Araujo, Amy B. O'Donnell, John B. McKinlay, "The Relationship between Libido and Testosterone Levels in Aging Men," *The Journal of Clinical Endocrinology & Metabolism*, Volume 91, Issue 7, 1 July 2006: 2509–2513, https://doi.org/10.1210/jc.2005-2508.

214   *Oxford Living Dicrionaries*, s.v., "Cognition," accessed January 9, 2019, https://en.oxforddictionaries.com/definition/cognition.

cognition. [215,216] In one study, 40 patients were treated for prostate cancer for 36 weeks through chemical castration—a process by which subjects take drugs to reduce androgens (male sex hormones) in the body. Doesn't sound pleasant, does it? The theory is that a reduction in androgens can potentially ward off prostate cancer. Whoever came up with that bright idea?

After this initial period, subjects were monitored for an additional 18 weeks. Interestingly, the researchers saw improvements in cognitive function and word recall only *after* treatment was stopped— suggesting once androgen concentrations increased, so did their memory.

One two-year study followed 19 males who received testosterone replacement therapy. The researchers noted improved attention, visual scanning ability, working memory and psychomotor ability (i.e., the ability to process tasks).[217] And one interesting placebo-controlled study involved 106 men with total testosterone below 330 ng/dL (11.4 nmol/L). The testosterone group was given 1,000 mg of testosterone undecanoate (Nebido/Aveed) injections every three months. And in those who had poor cognition before receiving testosterone, the researchers observed significant cognitive improvement.

215    Cappa SF, Guariglia C, Papagno C, Pizzamiglio L, Vallar G, Zoccolotti P, Ambrosi B, Santiemma V, "Effects of Testosterone Therapy on Cognitive Function in Aging: A Systematic Review," *Cogn Behav Neurol*, 2016 Sep, 29(3): 122–38, doi: 10.1097/WNN.0000000000000104.

216    Beauchet, O, "Testosterone and cognitive function: current clinical evidence of a relationship," *J Androl*, 2003 Jul–Aug, 24(4): 568–76.

217    Lašaitė L, Čeponis J, Preikša RT, Žilaitienė B, "Effects of two-year testosterone replacement therapy on cognition, emotions and quality of life in young and middle-aged hypogonadal men," *Andrologia*, 2017 Apr, 49(3), doi: 10.1111/and.12633.

## TESTOSTERONE AND THE HEART

Your heart is responsible for pumping blood throughout your body, and is working 24/7 on your behalf to keep you alive, so its importance cannot be overstated. However, few people appreciate the role of hormones—particularly testosterone—to heart health. And if anything, they believe it to be harmful! Although research shows low testosterone is actually detrimental to the heart. Studies show a *statistically significant* association between low testosterone, increased cardiovascular disease, and all-cause mortality.[218] In other words, low testosterone can lead to a heart attack!

In contrast, research shows higher concentrations of testosterone are linked with lower cardiovascular risk, improved cardiovascular risk factors, and reduced mortality in men who undergo testosterone therapy.[219] This is illustrated further by a seven-year control study on 2,314 men, age 40–79 years. After adjusting for parameters such as smoking and obesity, researchers found that every 173 ng/dL (6 nmol/L) increase in serum testosterone was associated with a 21% lower risk of all-cause mortality.[220] It's no coincidence then that deaths from cardiovascular disease have risen 41% between 1990 and

---

218   Amos Tambo, Mohsin H.K. Roshan, and Nikolai P. Pace, "Testosterone and Cardiovascular Disease," *Open Cardiovasc Med J*, 2016, 10: 1–10, published online 2016 Jan 15, doi: 10.2174/1874192401610010001.

219   Travis Goodale, M.D., Archana Sadhu, M.D., Steven Petak, M.D., J.D., and Richard Robbins, M.D., "Testosterone and the Heart," *Methodist Debakey Cardiovasc J*, 2017 Apr–Jun, 13(2): 68–72, doi: 10.14797/mdcj-13-2-68.

220   Khaw KT, Dowsett M, Folkerd E, Bingham S, Wareham N, Luben R, Welch A, Day N, "Endogenous testosterone and mortality due to all causes, cardiovascular disease, and cancer in men: European prospective investigation into cancer in Norfolk," (EPIC-Norfolk) *Prospective Population Study*, Circulation, 2007 Dec 4, 116(23): 2694–701.

2013,[221] while at the same time we are witnessing a global epidemic of low testosterone.

This idea that testosterone is bad for the heart appears to stem from the observational link between sudden death and anabolic steroid abuse in athletes. And now this line of thought has somehow made its way into mainstream and medical thinking with therapeutic testosterone. However, according to researchers, there appears to be no significant link in the literature between adverse cardiovascular events (i.e., heart attacks) and anabolic steroids and, by extension, testosterone. In fact, it's the chronic use of high-dose anabolic steroids that lead to death.[222] And as you've already seen from the chapter on anabolic steroids, there is a WORLD of difference between therapeutic testosterone and massive anabolic doses taken by bodybuilders. When it comes to testosterone and heart health, you have nothing to fear but everything to gain!

## TESTOSTERONE AND BONE HEALTH

Strong bones are essential for health, and they store important minerals such as calcium and phosphorous. And when they are required for use by the body, these minerals are then released into the bloodstream. In men, bone loss begins in the mid-30s and is associated with low concentrations of sex hormones.[223] You may think weak bones are only a concern for the elderly—but strong

---

221   Gregory A. Roth, M.D. et al. "Demographic and Epidemiologic Drivers of Global Cardiovascular Mortality," *N Engl J Med*, 2015, 372: 1333–41, DOI: 10.1056/ NEJMoa1406656.

222   Amos Tambo, Mohsin H.K. Roshan, and Nikolai P. Pace, "Testosterone and Cardiovascular Disease," *Open Cardiovasc Med J*, 2016, 10: 1–10, published online 2016 Jan 15, doi: 10.2174/1874192401610010001.

223   Bonny L Specker, Howard E Wey, and Eric P Smith, "Rates of bone loss in young adult males," *Int J Clin Rheumtol*, 2010 Apr 1, 5(2): 215–228, doi: 10.2217/ ijr.10.7.

bones also prevent against injury and fracture. Indeed, I've seen several young guys suffer bone injuries and fractures from contact sports that could have been avoided. Because their bones were so frail, they were much more susceptible. Indeed, I believe the issue of weak bones among the young population has largely gone unnoticed by mainstream society.

Multiple studies show a link between low serum testosterone concentrations and low bone mineral density in young and old men alike.[224,225] Once more, we can look at the effect of androgen deprivation therapy on men with prostate cancer as an example of what happens when testosterone is taken away. Multiple studies show osteoporosis (bone loss) as a negative side effect of androgen deprivation therapy—highlighting the importance of testosterone to bone health.[226,227] One study looked at the effect of hypogonadism on calcium and bone density on 11 young men with an average age of 23. The authors concluded that low testosterone, even for a short time, can have a **"profound negative effect"** on calcium and bone metabolism.[228]

224    Katznelson L, Finkelstein JS, Schoenfeld DA, Rosenthal DI, Anderson EJ, Klibanski A, "Increase in bone density and lean body mass during testosterone administration in men with acquired hypogonadism," *J Clin Endocrinol Metab*, 1996 Dec, 81(12): 4358–65.

225    Canale D, Vignali E, Golia F, Martino E, Pinchera A, Marcocci C, Katznelson L, Finkelstein JS, Schoenfeld DA, Rosenthal DI, Anderson EJ, Klibanski A, "Effects of hormonal replacement treatment on bone mineral density and metabolism in hypogonadal patients," *Mol Cell Endocrinol*, 2000 Mar 30, 161(1–2): 47–51.

226    Ross RW, Small EJ, "Osteoporosis in men treated with androgen deprivation therapy for prostate cancer," *J Urol*, 2002 May, 167(5): 1952–6.

227    Diamond TH, Higano CS, Smith MR, Guise TA, Singer FR, "Osteoporosis in men with prostate carcinoma receiving androgen-deprivation therapy: recommendations for diagnosis and therapies," *Cancer*, 2004 Mar 1, 100(5): 892–9.

228    Mauras N, Hayes VY, Vieira NE, Yergey AL, O'Brien KO, "Profound hypogonadism has significant negative effects on calcium balance in males: a calcium kinetic study," *J Bone Miner Res*, 1999 Apr, 14(4): 577–82.

Although it appears it's not only low serum testosterone concentrations but also low estradiol concentrations that are responsible for poor bone health.[229,230] And as we'll see later, estradiol, a form of estrogen, is fundamental to male health.

Several studies show testosterone therapy improves bone mineral density in men.[231,232] In one double-blind study, 108 hypogonadal men age 65 were given either a testosterone patch or placebo for 36 months. The researchers didn't see much change in lumbar spine bone health in men whose testosterone levels were the equivalent of mid-range for younger men, but they saw it improve in men with low pretreatment serum testosterone.[233]

As we can see from this chapter, the overwhelming evidence is that testosterone is a net positive for your health. If you've followed the advice from previous chapters, and it turns out you need to take testosterone, then now you can rest assured it's not the monster it's made out to be. Of course, I am not going to sit here and claim

---

229    Gary Golds, Devon Houdek, and Terra Arnason. "Male Hypogonadism and Osteoporosis: The Effects, Clinical Consequences, and Treatment of Testosterone Deficiency in Bone Health," *International Journal of Endocrinology*, Volume 2017 (2017), Article ID 4602129, 15 pages, https://doi.org/10.1155/2017/4602129.

230    Nur-Vaizura Mohamad, Ima-Nirwana Soelaiman, and Kok-Yong Chin, "A concise review of testosterone and bone health," *Clin Interv Aging*, 2016, 11: 1317–1324, published online 2016 Sep 22, doi: 10.2147/CIA.S115472.

231    Pierre M.G. Bouloux et al., "Effects of oral testosterone undecanoate therapy on bone mineral density and body composition in 322 aging men with symptomatic testosterone deficiency: a 1-year, randomized, placebo-controlled, dose-ranging study," *The Aging Male*, Volume 16, 2013, Issue 2.

232    J. Rodriguez-Tolrà, J. Torremadé, S. di Gregorio, L. del Rio, E. Franco, "Effects of testosterone treatment on bone mineral density in men with testosterone deficiency syndrome," *American Society of Andrology and European Academy of Andrology*, 20 May 2013, https://doi.org/10.1111/j.2047-2927.2013.00090.x.

233    Snyder, PJ et al., "Effect of testosterone treatment on bone mineral density in men over 65 years of age," *J Clin Endocrinol Metab*, 1999 Jun, 84(6): 1966–72.

that it's all roses and there are no side effects. However, the side effects of treatment with testosterone can be mitigated if not avoided altogether with a proper protocol. And in the following chapter, I'll show you how to do just that.

# CHAPTER 11

# TESTOSTERONE REPLACEMENT THERAPY PROTOCOLS

By now you understand the importance of testosterone to the health and well-being of every man. And with the constant barrage of testosterone-lowering substances in our environment, it's any wonder we have testosterone at all. Perhaps you've had no joy increasing your testosterone levels, despite following many of the strategies discussed in this book. I encourage you to exhaust all tools at your disposal before you resort to testosterone replacement therapy. Nevertheless, it's possible your low testosterone is a medical issue that requires treatment. Testosterone replacement therapy is cutting-edge, so it's vital you understand the available treatment options. Why? Because many physicians do not understand it themselves; therefore, you must educate yourself about it.

Should young men be treated differently to older men with regard to testosterone replacement therapy? The answer is yes and no. While men are often capable of fathering children well into middle age, men under 35 years old are considered to be of prime childbearing age. Many doctors, for reasons we'll go into, are hesitant to put young men on TRT. Doctors often refuse to treat them because they "shouldn't have to worry about testosterone" at their age. However, age should not be a barrier to treatment for low testosterone, and when you have symptoms, they should be treated. In this chapter, we will cover the fundamentals of testosterone replacement therapy so you can undergo treatment the right way.

## TESTOSTERONE INJECTIONS, CREAMS, AND GELS

Today, several treatment options exist for TRT. These include injections, creams, gels, lozenges, pellets, buccal (oral patch), and—more recently—nasal spray has emerged as a potential option. However, for the purposes of this book we will focus on injections, creams, and gels. They represent the best options for testosterone therapy due to their ability to elevate serum testosterone to optimal levels in a predictable and consistent manner.[234]

## INJECTIONS

Testosterone injections (shots) are seen as gold standard for testosterone replacement therapy. Although, as we'll see shortly, there's evidence to suggest scrotal application of creams is the optimal treatment protocol.

Above all, ensure testosterone goes directly into the bloodstream, and the result is an elevation of serum testosterone in a stable and predictable fashion. Injectable forms of testosterone (e.g., enanthate, Sustanon, propionate, etc.) are suspended in oil preparations known as *esters*.

Esters lower the water solubility of a steroid and are designed to accomplish one thing: to slow the release of the testosterone into the bloodstream. Without the ester, pure testosterone by itself would be metabolized (i.e., processed) by the body in under five hours, meaning you would have to inject several times a day. As we'll see in a moment, depending on the ester, testosterone can be released steadily into the bloodstream anywhere from two days to twelve weeks.

---

234   Kishore M Lakshman and Shehzad Basaria, "Safety and efficacy of testosterone gel in the treatment of male hypogonadism," *Clin Interv Aging*, 2009, 4: 397–412.

I often hear stories about how guys feel different on one type of testosterone ester over another. For example, "I feel much better taking enanthate instead of Sustanon!" But in the end, testosterone is testosterone—and there isn't really any difference between them. It's the dose and frequency of injection that are the determining factors—not the type of ester involved. Author William Llewellyn sums it up, "Your muscle cells see only testosterone; ultimately there is no difference. Reports of varying issues of muscle gain, androgenic side effects, water retention, etc. are only issues of timing."[235]

The downside of injectables is that you actually have to inject! Indeed, the idea of inserting a foreign object into your body doesn't come naturally. And this disqualifies many guys from injections altogether, as it isn't easy to overcome this trepidation. In addition, injections require more preparation and effort because you have to dispose of the medical supplies (i.e., glass vials, ampoules, and needles). But once you're used to it, this is relatively straightforward.

## TESTOSTERONE INJECTIONS: THE OPTIMAL TREATMENT PROTOCOL

Below are the most common of injectable testosterone options used for testosterone replacement therapy.

### TESTOSTERONE ENANTHATE AND CYPIONATE

Testosterone enanthate is a long-acting single ester injectable that has a half-life of approximately eight days. "Half-life" means the amount of time it takes for a drug to be reduced to half its initial value in your body. The compound derives its name from the carboxylic acid ester known as enanthate that is attached to the testosterone hormone.

---

235   Llewellyn, *ANABOLICS*.

Testosterone cypionate is another long-acting single ester compound. As with enanthate, the half-life for cypionate is also eight days, making them almost identical. Although, cypionate differs due to the carboxylic acid ester that the testosterone solution is held in.

Enanthate is widely available throughout the world, and in many countries is the primary injectable compound for testosterone therapy. Cypionate is common in the US but not so much in Europe.

## TESTOSTERONE PROPIONATE

Testosterone propionate was developed in the 1930s and was one of the original testosterone compounds—and it still remains popular today. It is a short-acting, single ester compound with a half-life of around four days.

This short-acting ester means you require frequent injections. In the eyes of many people, this is an advantage because it closely mimics the body's natural testosterone production.

Due to the increased injection frequency with propionate— sometimes every other day—many prefer longer-acting esters such as enanthate over propionate. It is still widely used in the US, but rarely in Europe, where longer-acting esters are more favored.

## TESTOSTERONE UNDECANOATE

Testosterone undecanoate, also known by its trade names Nebido and Aveed, is an extremely long-acting ester. Some manufacturers state undecanoate has a half-life of 90 days, although research suggests the half-life may be closer to 34 days.[236] A typical injection

---

236   Behre HM, Abshagen K, Oettel M, Hübler D, Nieschlag E, "Intramuscular injection of testosterone undecanoate for the treatment of male hypogonadism: phase I studies," *Eur J Endocrinol*, 1999 May, 140(5): 414–9.

protocol for undecanoate would be 1,000 mg every 10–14 weeks, and some doctors may do as frequent as every eight weeks.

The main benefit of testosterone undecanoate is that it requires fewer injections. But in practice, most men don't have a good experience with undecanoate. The initial dose is quite substantial and may provide relief of symptoms for a few weeks. However, the effects start to subside after that early period because testosterone levels start to drop, meaning it can be a long wait until the next injection. I've known several instances where men have switched to a shorter ester such as Sustanon or enanthate because of the roller-coaster ride with undecanoate.

## SUSTANON

Sustanon, also known as Sustanon 250, is an oil-based injectable consisting of four different testosterone esters: testosterone propionate (30 mg), testosterone phenylpropionate (60 mg), testosterone isocaproate (60 mg), and testosterone decanoate (100 mg).

Sustanon injections were originally developed for patients to receive the fast-acting benefits of testosterone over an extended period. The idea of using a combination of short- and long-duration esters was for people to be able to inject every 2–3 weeks.

This sounds great in practice. Fewer injections means less hassle, right? Sadly not. This type of injection frequency inevitably produces what Sustanon was meant to prevent: Peaks and valleys in blood testosterone levels.

The manufacturer of Sustanon produces it in glass ampoules. As a result, they are not as straightforward to use as the multi-dose vials seen in the US. It does take some practice, but it's simple once you learn how to do it.

To learn how to open glass ampoules, you can check out this video on YouTube:

https://www.youtube.com/watch?v=3l9p4VXVaOk

I watched this video before I opened my first ampoule. Needless to say, I applied too much pressure and broke several ampoules before I got it right. But to avoid going through this process in the first place, I recommend you simply purchase a glass ampoule-opener.

INJECTION DOSAGE: Testosterone replacement therapy is still on the cutting edge of medical science. At this moment in time, there are no "industry accepted" practices for dosages and frequency, and prescriptions can vary from one doctor to the next.

Unfortunately, when it comes to TRT, many physicians still abide by outdated textbook practices. As a result, they use protocols that recommend patients inject every 2–3 weeks. Doctors who prescribe in this manner fail to grasp the basics of pharmacokinetics (i.e., how long the testosterone remains in the bloodstream).

If they did, they would realize injections of 2–3 weeks are wholly inadequate, resulting in a very unpleasant experience for the patient—from feeling good after the initial injection, to feeling anxious, lethargic, and suffering low sex drive only a week or so later because the concentration of testosterone in their bloodstream is markedly reduced. However, given the dogmatic adherence to textbooks and outdated practices, I don't see this changing anytime soon.

Progressive physicians like Dr. Merrill Matschke, Dr. John Crisler, and Dr. Keith Nichols understand that frequent injections, typically anywhere from daily to twice a week, result in the best experience for the patient. This type of injection frequency means blood testosterone levels are consistently maintained within the optimal range.

Maintaining consistent levels of blood testosterone means patients experience the full benefits of treatment (i.e., improved mood, libido, etc.). This avoids the side effects that occur due to a drop-off in testosterone levels. I cannot overemphasize the importance of finding a competent doctor, and we'll discuss this in the next chapter.

After consulting with hundreds of men on hormonal balance and TRT, the optimum protocol for most tends to be 100–200 mg of injectable, intramuscular testosterone, every 3.5 days. In my experience, this strikes the balance between maintaining a stable level of blood testosterone, while minimizing injection frequency. This works well with long-acting esters such as enanthate, cypionate, and Sustanon, whereas propionate requires more frequent injections due to the shorter ester.

You could optimize even further by injecting more frequently. But that means you would have to inject either daily or every other day. And for most men, that's far too often. For further guidance on advanced injection protocols, I recommend you read Jay Campbell's book *The Testosterone Optimization Therapy Bible*.

## CREAMS AND GELS

For many men, transdermal creams and gels are a favored form of testosterone treatment and are ideal for men apprehensive of injections. They're simple to use; you apply the solution to your skin once or twice daily then go about your business. In addition, creams and gels require no special training or instruction for use. However, this type of treatment does not come without its drawbacks.

One disadvantage of transdermals is the poor absorption through skin. According to Dr. John Crisler, this is because the delivery of transdermal testosterone is through blood vessels in the skin, and this transportation process means less testosterone is absorbed (in comparison to injectables).[237] Due to this poor absorption, gels and creams often fail to elevate serum testosterone levels to the optimal range.

Time and again, I've seen men use transdermal creams, only to have average testosterone levels and feel merely okay. Why undergo a lifelong treatment just to feel okay? Admittedly, I used to think this was because transdermals were flawed as a treatment option. However, that was until I spoke with Dr. Keith Nichols, a leading hormone optimization physician, who argues that transdermals themselves are not the problem. It's their application and concentration that's the issue (i.e., how and where they are applied, and how much testosterone is used).

Androgel is one of the most popular topical gels used for TRT and comes in a 1% or 1.62% concentration. This is typically applied to the shoulders, upper arms, or abdominal area—but not to the scrotum, as it contains alcohol. The low concentration of testosterone and poor absorption of gels means more needs to be applied to a larger surface area, which makes it quite inefficient. And because you have to use so much gel just to get an effect, treatment can become expensive.

According to Dr. Nichols, transdermal cream application to the scrotum is superior to both gels and injectables, and he himself has used this method with great success in his practice. Transdermal creams are able to hold a greater concentration of testosterone in comparison to gels. This leads to greater success in elevating blood testosterone into the optimal range. And in the interview with Dr. Nichols later in the book, we'll see what "optimal" really means.

Transdermal creams applied to the scrotum can also elevate DHT levels, due to the expression of the 5-alpha reductase enzyme in

---

237    Campbell, *The Testosterone Optimization Therapy Bible.*

the skin (responsible for converting testosterone to DHT). This can dramatically improve libido and erectile function, as DHT has been shown to play a key role in male sexual function.[238]

In addition, one key benefits of transdermal creams application to the scrotum is that it does not typically result in estrogenic side effects such as nipple tenderness or water retention, as is often the case with injectables. Dr. Nichols also points out that injectable testosterone can lower HDL (good cholesterol) in some patients, due to the metabolization (processing) of the ester solution by the liver.

CREAMS DOSAGE: It's not recommended you use a gel application for TRT due to poor absorption and low testosterone concentration. Dr. Keith Nichols recommends using a 20% concentration (200 mg per gram) testosterone cream. It's important that it contains no alcohol, as alcohol can burn the skin on the scrotum. His protocol involves applying 100 mg of cream to the scrotum twice a day—once in the morning and once in the evening.

There are a few things to note with this protocol. First, the area of the scrotum must be clean, shaven, and dry prior to application to ensure maximal absorption through the skin. Showering, swimming, and exercise must be avoided for up to four hours after application so the cream can absorb properly. In addition, you must avoid sexual contact with your partner to prevent transference of the cream before it dries.

---

238   Abdulmaged M. Traish, Ashwini Mulgaonkar, Nicholas Giordano, "The Dark Side of 5α-Reductase Inhibitors' Therapy: Sexual Dysfunction, High Gleason Grade Prostate Cancer and Depression," *Korean J Urol*, 2014 Jun, 55(6): 367–379, published online 2014 Jun 16, doi: 10.4111/kju.2014.55.6.367.

THE BENEFITS: We've already spoken at length on the benefits of testosterone in the book, but to summarize, here they are:

- Increased muscle mass and strength
- Increased insulin sensitivity
- Improved sexual desire
- Improved mood and energy
- Improved cognition[239]

As far as I'm concerned, using testosterone is the number one way to reap all the benefits of hormone optimization. I've seen Clomid and hCG monotherapy (discussed in a moment) work well in many men. However, in my experience, you don't get the full spectrum of benefits with these treatments the way you do with testosterone. And while the patient may feel good on Clomid or hCG, sometimes they struggle consistently with certain aspects, such as libido.

SIDE EFFECTS: The side effects of testosterone can be broken down into two main categories: Estrogenic (from estrogen) and androgenic (from androgens, or male sex hormones).

**Estrogenic.** These side effects occur due to too much estrogen and include:

- Water retention
- Puffiness
- Bloating
- Sensitive nipples
- Gynecomastia
- Moodiness
- Poor erection quality

---

239    Nazem Bassil, Saad Alkaade, and John E Morley, "The benefits and risks of testosterone replacement therapy: a review," *Ther Clin Risk Manag*, 2009, 5: 427–448, published online 2009 Jun 22.

**Androgenic.** These are "masculinizing" side effects and include:

- Acne
- Oily skin
- Male pattern baldness (in those genetically predisposed)
- Body and facial hair growth

In addition to the above, testosterone stimulates red blood cell production, which can raise hematocrit levels (HCT). Hematocrit is a volume percentage measure of total red blood cells. Most doctors monitor HCT levels closely with TRT because it was thought a high red blood cell count could lead to a stroke. As a result, physicians often order patients to take therapeutic phlebotomies (blood draw) to reduce red blood cell count. However, subsequent research has revealed elevations in hemoglobin and hematocrit levels from testosterone therapy are actually benign,[240] much like a Kenyan long-distance runner has a high red blood cell count from living at altitude.

One drawback or side effect of using transdermal creams and gels is the need to avoid water and exercise (albeit temporarily), as well as contact with sexual partners to prevent transference of the testosterone. Whereas with injections, this is not an issue, as the testosterone goes directly into the bloodstream.

## CLOMID

Clomiphene citrate, also known as Clomid, is a selective estrogen receptor modulator (SERM). SERMs are a class of compounds that act on estrogen receptors by blocking the action of estrogen. Clomid works by blocking the action of estrogen in the pituitary gland (i.e., the part of the brain that secretes gonadotropins). As a result of this

---

240  Campbell, *The Testosterone Optimization Therapy Bible.*

blocking action, the pituitary detects less estrogen and responds by secreting luteinizing hormone (LH).

Clomid has been in use since the 1960s to stimulate ovulation in women. More recently, it has been used as an off-label medication to treat secondary hypogonadism and male infertility.[241] Today it has become increasingly adopted by physicians to treat hypogonadism, particularly for young men who wish to restore their testosterone levels while maintaining fertility.

The research on Clomid use in young men is promising. One study monitored 89 men age 22–37 undergoing treatment for hypogonadism with Clomid. Testosterone and gonadotropin levels (i.e., FSH and LH) were measured prior to and during treatment. The majority of men (70%) took 25 mg every other day (EOD), while the remaining took 50 mg EOD. Researchers noted a significant increase in testosterone and gonadotropin levels, and more than half the patients saw an improvement in at least three symptoms of low testosterone. Interestingly, there were also no major side effects noted.[242]

In my experience, the success of Clomid as a remedy for low testosterone is subjective and depends on the individual. Some men feel fantastic on Clomid; reporting improved sex drive, mood, and overall sense of well-being. Comparatively, other men feel terrible on it and fail to see significant improvement in their symptoms, while reporting feelings of moodiness, bloating, and lack of energy. With Clomid, it's often a case of trying it to see if it works for you. If it

241   Ranjith Ramasamy, Joseph M Armstrong, and Larry I Lipshultz, "Preserving fertility in the hypogonadal patient: an update," *Asian J Androl*, 2015 Mar–Apr, 17(2): 197–200, published online 2014 Oct 3, doi: 10.4103/1008-682X.142772.

242   Katz DJ, Nabulsi O, Tal R, Mulhall JP, "Outcomes of clomiphene citrate treatment in young hypogonadal men," *BJU Int*, 2012 Aug, 110(4): 573–8, doi: 10.1111/j.1464-410X.2011.10702.x.

doesn't, you can always move on to alternative treatment protocol (e.g., testosterone replacement).

## CLOMID: THE OPTIMAL TREATMENT PROTOCOL

DOSAGE: Forward-thinking doctors such as Dr. Rob Kominiarek and Dr. John Crisler favor using 12.5 mg to 25 mg of Clomid every other day with their patients to restore testosterone production and maintain fertility. I have heard of some physicians prescribing 25 mg to 50 mg every day. This is far too much and will usually result in unwanted side effects. While this dose may result in elevations of serum testosterone, it will typically also lead to high levels of SHBG and estradiol that counteract the positive effects of testosterone.

THE BENEFITS: There are a couple of standout benefits of Clomid. First, the barrier to entry is low—as it doesn't get any simpler than taking a pill. Second, it is one of the least invasive forms of treatment and doesn't shut down your endogenous testosterone production.

Clomid has the potential to maintain fertility AND elevate your testosterone levels, meaning you don't need to take multiple medications. By raising your serum testosterone levels to the optimal end of the normal range, you should receive all the benefits of testosterone replacement therapy. And another thing to note is that, of all the treatment options discussed in this chapter, Clomid is the cheapest.

SIDE EFFECTS: The side effects profile of Clomid tends to mirror those of testosterone. Although in some men, Clomid can elevate SHBG levels, resulting in less free or bioavailable testosterone. So with less free testosterone, the patient is unlikely to receive the benefits of treatment, despite higher concentrations of serum testosterone. Clomid can also cause elevations of estrogen, resulting in water retention, moodiness, puffiness, and poor erection quality.

The consensus is that Clomid's half-life is between 4–6 weeks. Anecdotally, however, I have seen men's blood markers to continue to be affected by Clomid, despite the fact they stopped taking it several weeks prior. There have also been some reports of Clomid causing vision problems in some individuals, including blurred vision and flashing lights. This is thought to happen because Clomid can have an antagonistic effect on the estrogen receptors in the pituitary. Nonetheless, this appears to be a rare occurrence among Clomid users.

## hCG

Human chorionic gonadotropin, also known as hCG, is a hormone produced in different levels in both men and women. HCG was originally identified as a hormone produced in the female placenta. HCG shares a similar molecular structure to luteinizing hormone (LH). This means that when taken, it behaves in a similar manner to LH in the male body. If you recall, LH is secreted by the pituitary gland to stimulate production of testosterone in the testes. Therefore, as hCG mirrors the action of LH, injecting sends a signal to the testes to produce testosterone.[243]

The main benefit of using hCG is that it keeps the hypothalamic pituitary axis (HPTA) intact by stimulating endogenous testosterone production. This means patients using hCG are able to maintain fertility. HCG is recommended for men who want to father children, while receiving the benefits of optimal testosterone levels.

Clinical studies demonstrate that hCG is effective at maintaining intratesticular (i.e., natural) testosterone levels and maintaining sperm levels. In one randomized control study of 29 healthy males,

243    Jeffrey Dach, MD, "John Crisler on How to Use HCG in Males with Low Testosterone," Jeffrey Dach MD, June 24, 2013, https://jeffreydachmd.com/2013/11/john-crisler-hcg-males-low-testosterone/

200 mg of testosterone enanthate was injected alongside either a placebo or 125, 250, 500 IU dose of hCG every other day.

Compared to average baseline serum testosterone levels of 400 ng/dL (14.1 nmol/L), intratesticular levels in the testosterone-only group were suppressed 94%, 25% in the 125 IU group, 7% in the 250 IU group, while they increased 26% in the 500 IU hCG group.[244]

Some men may not want children at the time of undergoing testosterone replacement therapy but may want them in the future. As a result, they may opt for exogenous testosterone (i.e., TRT) until they are ready to father children. However, in any case, hCG would still be advised alongside in order to maintain integrity of sperm production pathways.

HCG can be used in conjunction with testosterone or as a monotherapy (i.e., by itself). Patients typically only undergo treatment with hCG as a monotherapy if they have secondary hypogonadism (i.e., due to a problem with signaling from the hypothalamus or pituitary).

However, an individual with primary hypogonadism—where the testes fail to respond to signals sent from the brain to stimulate testosterone production—would be unsuited to hCG monotherapy. This is because, even though the signal to produce testosterone (created by hCG) is sent to the testes, they will fail to respond regardless.

## hCG: THE OPTIMAL TREATMENT PROTOCOL

<u>DOSAGE:</u> The hCG dose depends on the treatment protocol used. Is the patient using hCG as a standalone monotherapy to optimize testosterone and maintain fertility? Or is it used conjunction with

---

244    Ranjith Ramasamy, Joseph M Armstrong, and Larry I Lipshultz, "Preserving fertility in the hypogonadal patient: an update," *Asian J Androl*, 2015 Mar–Apr, 17(2): 197–200, published online 2014 Oct 3, doi: 10.4103/1008-682X.142772.

testosterone to maintain fertility? Each treatment protocol will require a difference approach.

Most physicians who prescribe hCG tend to use it in conjunction with testosterone, and its use as a monotherapy is less widespread. As such, there is limited data on hCG as a monotherapy. One study looked at the effect of 3,000 IU hCG every other day (EOD) on fertility levels of 49 men who had previously taken exogenous testosterone. In total, 47 men (95.9%) saw a return of fertility, with one man documenting pregnancy without follow-up semen analysis.[245]

In practice, 1,500 IU of hCG injected subcutaneously (i.e., into fat tissue) is standard protocol when it's used as a standalone therapy. Although, subjectively, some men may feel better at 3,000 IU EOD, as per the above study.

Regarding the use of hCG alongside TRT, research and anecdotal evidence suggest an optimal dose of 500 IU EOD—or 1,500 IU per week. This appears to strike the balance between the positive effects of testosterone, while minimizing estrogenic side effects that can occur with the addition of hCG. This is because hCG will raise intratesticular testosterone (alongside the inclusion of exogenous testosterone), leading to the elevated estrogen levels. A typical injection protocol for 500 IU EOD hCG may be Monday, Wednesday, Friday, with testosterone injections on Tuesday and Saturday. **NOTE:** hCG is injected subcutaneously (i.e., into belly fat tissue), while testosterone is typically injected intramuscularly.

One study evaluated the effect of 500 IU hCG EOD on men undergoing TRT. There were 26 men with an average age of 35.9

---

245   Wenker EP, Dupree JM, Langille GM, Kovac J, Ramasamy R, Lamb D, Mills JN, Lipshultz LI, "The Use of HCG-Based Combination Therapy for Recovery of Spermatogenesis after Testosterone Use," *J Sex Med*, 2015 Jun, 12(6): 1334–7, doi: 10.1111/jsm.12890. Epub 2015 Apr 22.

years who took part in the study. After one year, none of the men were infertile, and no impact was observed on semen parameters, and 9 out of 26 were able to conceive with their partners.[246]

BENEFITS: The benefit of hCG is the ability to elevate testosterone levels while maintaining fertility. Improved endogenous (i.e., made from the body) testosterone provides the same benefits to your health in a similar manner to testosterone replacement therapy. Although in my experience, some of the effects of hCG tend to be more subtle in comparison to exogenous testosterone. For example, you may experience an increase in lean body mass while on hCG, though it's not clear whether hCG improves strength in the same manner as exogenous testosterone.[247]

SIDE EFFECTS: The side effects of hCG tend to be more estrogenic, as opposed to androgenic with testosterone. They include water retention, bloating, gynecomastia, and loss of libido. Although it should be noted, as with testosterone, these side effects can mostly be mitigated through correct dosing and injection frequency.

## "DO I NEED TO TAKE AN AI?"

Aromatase inhibitors (AIs) were originally developed to treat conditions such as breast cancer and gynecomastia. And today their application has also extended to testosterone replacement therapy. AIs inhibit the production of estrogen by blocking the activity of the aromatase enzyme, which is responsible for the conversion of

246   Hsieh TC, Pastuszak AW, Hwang K, Lipshultz LI, "Concomitant intramuscular human chorionic gonadotropin preserves spermatogenesis in men undergoing testosterone replacement therapy," *J Urol*, 2013 Feb, 189(2): 647–50, doi: 10.1016/j. juro.2012.09.043.

247   Shehzad Basaria, "Androgen Abuse in Athletes: Detection and Consequences," *The Journal of Clinical Endocrinology & Metabolism*, Volume 95, Issue 4, 1 April 2010: 1533–1543, https://doi.org/10.1210/jc.2009-1579.

androgens into estrogen. AIs are classed into two categories based on their chemical structure: steroidal and non-steroidal. The most common AIs are: exemestane (Aromasin)—a steroidal AI—and letrozole (Femara) and anastrozole (Arimidex)—both of which are non-steroidal.

Physicians tend to prescribe AIs alongside TRT because testosterone can cause estrogen levels to rise, resulting in unwanted estrogenic side effects, such as water retention and gynecomastia. Therefore, in order to treat and mitigate these side effects and avoid litigation, doctors tend to prescribe AIs as standard from the beginning.

On the surface this appears to be a prudent measure, but in recent times this practice has come under scrutiny because many doctors prescribe them too readily based on inaccurate blood tests that over-estimate estradiol levels (as discussed in chapter 3). The reason this is a problem is because they often prescribe excessive doses (e.g., 0.5 mg every other day), leading to unwanted side effects, such as bone mineral loss, erectile dysfunction, and low libido.

Ideally, AIs should be avoided altogether; if anything, for the simple fact you should minimize the amount of medications you take. What's more, these medications were never intended to be used by men in the long-term. So it's fair to say that we don't fully appreciate their long-term effects. As discussed in the interview with Dr. John Crisler, in many instances, over-the-counter supplements such as DIM and calcium-d-glucarate can be used to balance estrogen levels.

Leading hormone optimization physician Dr. Merrill Matschke always prefers to use nutraceuticals (i.e., food or nutrient supplements with medicinal benefits, derived from natural sources) over AIs. Dr. Matschke uses a supplement combining DIM, I3C, and calcium-d-glucarate to treat patients who experience high estrogen symptoms after undergoing TRT. He explains, though, that he will also prescribe this supplement for patients in the face of high estrogen levels even if they are asymptomatic. This prevents symptoms from developing in the first instance. Dr. Matschke will only use AIs as a last resort for patients who don't respond to nutraceuticals.

Men who see an elevation in estrogen after undergoing TRT tend to have high levels of body fat. This is because the aromatase enzyme is abundant in fat tissue, resulting in the excessive conversion of testosterone to estrogen. This is why it's so important to lead a testosterone-friendly lifestyle while on TRT—it's not just for men trying to raise their natural levels.

There are instances of men with low body fat that take testosterone but still end up with high levels of estrogen. I myself was one of these, even though my body fat levels stay well below 15% year round. Frankly, I was against taking AIs for a long-time, as I never really had any obvious symptoms of high estrogen, such as water retention, nipple swelling, etc. Eventually, I realized I often suffered dramatic mood swings and that this could be due to elevated estrogen levels.

Some days I would feel on top of the world, while others I wanted to go hide under a rock. I found myself getting teary-eyed and emotional over trivial things. In addition, my libido was not what it should have been for a 30-year-old man taking testosterone. So under the guidance of my doctor, I took a small 0.5 mg weekly dose of anastrozole.

As a result, my libido and erection quality improved. On an emotional level, I felt calmer and more relaxed than before. This experience taught me AIs may be warranted when there is a clinical need. However, after consulting with Dr. Crisler and Dr. Matschke, I will be experimenting with a DIM supplement going forward in an effort to reduce my reliance on multiple medications.

There is a lack of clinical data to suggest long-term AI use negatively affects men's health, and further research is required on this front. Some studies on rats and postmenopausal women suggest that the inhibition of estrogen production can lead to increased anxiety.[248,249] Therefore, we may conclude lowering estrogen will have a similar effect on men. There is evidence to show that the anxiety-lowering and antidepressant effect of testosterone is mediated by estrogen.[250] So by artificially lowering the amount of estrogen in the blood, you may counteract the positive effects of testosterone.

To summarize, it's clear long-term low levels of estrogen is not good for men. In summary, aim to use a DIM supplement before resorting to an AI. If your doctor does insist you take an AI, you should question it—especially if they want you to take it from the outset.

If your physician is doing their job properly, they should monitor the effect of testosterone therapy *before* prescribing an AI. Because if you use multiple medications all at once, how do you know the individual effect each one has? The answer is you don't. If you are prescribed an AI, aim to use the minimal effective dose (i.e., the smallest quantity possible for maximal effect). This dose is typically 0.25–0.5 mg every 5–7 days. (And, most importantly, refrain from using an AI until you suffer high E2 symptoms/side effects.)

---

248   Meng FT, Ni RJ, Zhang Z, Zhao J, Liu YJ, Zhou JN, "Inhibition of oestrogen biosynthesis induces mild anxiety in C57BL/6J ovariectomized female mice," *Neurosci Bull*, 2011 Aug, 27(4): 241–50, doi: 10.1007/s12264-011-1014-8.

249   Kelly Anne Phillips, Karin Ribi, and Richard Fisher, "Do aromatase inhibitors have adverse effects on cognitive function?" *Breast Cancer Res*, 2011, 13(1): 203, doi: 10.1186/bcr2806.

250   Nicole Carrier, Samantha K. Saland, Florian Duclot, Huan He, Roger Mercer, and Mohamed Kabbaj, "The Anxiolytic and Antidepressant-like Effects of Testosterone and Estrogen in Gonadectomized Male Rats," *Biol Psychiatry*, 2015 Aug 15, 78(4): 259–269, doi: 10.1016/j.biopsych.2014.12.024.

# THE IMPORTANCE OF ESTROGEN

You already understand the importance of testosterone to male health—now it's time to understand the importance estrogen as well. There is a pervading myth that estrogen is bad for male health. This idea comes from bodybuilding, where taking massive amounts of anabolic steroids is the norm. These massive doses result in elevated estrogen levels, leading to side effects such as puffiness (moon face), water retention, decreased erectile function, and in some cases gynecomastia (bitch tits). Therefore, bodybuilders conclude estrogen is the devil incarnate. However, the problem is not estrogen but the ridiculous doses of anabolic steroids that elevate it in the first place.

This bodybuilding mentality has also spilled over to the hormone therapy space. Subsequently, one of the biggest concerns men have before undergoing TRT are estrogenic side effects. "Will I develop breasts?" "Will I become moody and bloated?" For the most part, though, their concerns are unfounded because anyone taking therapeutic doses of testosterone under the guidance of a competent physician will avoid estrogenic side effects.

Another common myth is that estrogen is somehow a "female hormone." The scary thing is, many doctors actually think this. I've had men tell me their doctor refused to test for estrogen because they consider it a female hormone. However, estrogen plays a vital role in male health. It is important for mood via its interaction with serotonin receptors in the brain, as well as cognition and emotional well-being.[251] It appears that estrogen may have a significant role in cognitive function, with aromatase receptors (to convert testosterone

---

251    Michael Schulster, Aaron M Bernie, Ranjith Ramasamy, "The role of estradiol in male reproductive function," *Asian Journal of Andrology* (2016) 18, 435–440.

into estrogen) found in key areas in the brain responsible for memory and learning, including the amygdala and hippocampus.[252]

In one study, 60 males age 50–90 years old were given 100 mg testosterone injection a week plus oral placebo, or 100 mg testosterone injection a week plus an oral aromatase inhibitor (i.e., to block or prevent the conversion of testosterone into estrogen). Spatial memory improved in both groups, but verbal memory only improved in those who didn't receive an aromatase inhibitor.[253] The results of the study suggest that estrogen plays an important role in verbal memory. It's important to note the patients were given an EXTREMELY high dose aromatase inhibitor—1 mg daily—a dose that *significantly* reduces estrogen levels. Thankfully, most doctors do not prescribe AIs in such large doses.

Hopefully, now you see why you shouldn't buy into the bro myth that estrogen is bad, nor is it a female hormone. Too much estrogen can have a detrimental effect on sexual function and well-being. But arbitrarily suppressing your estrogen with aromatase inhibitors because your doctor thinks it's the "right thing to do" is not an intelligent approach either. With estrogen, the reality is that it's a balancing act of where you feel best, and not a case of "chasing lab numbers" as many doctors tend to do. A good doctor should abide by the mantra "If it ain't broke, don't fix it." That is, in the absence of estrogenic symptoms, you should not take an AI.

252  Janowsky, JS, "Thinking with your gonads: testosterone and cognition," *Trends in Cognitive Sciences*, 2006, 10: 77–82.

253  Cherrier MM1, Matsumoto AM, Amory JK, Ahmed S, Bremner W, Peskind ER, Raskind MA, Johnson M, Craft S, "The role of aromatization in testosterone supplementation: effects on cognition in older men," *Neurology*, 2005 Jan 25, 64(2): 290–6.

## HOW LONG DOES IT TAKE TO FEEL THE EFFECTS OF TESTOSTERONE?

The million-dollar question: How long does it take to feel the effects of testosterone? Because of our unique biochemistry, this is a very individual thing, and it really depends on your starting point. For example, I've seen many guys who started out TRT with high SHBG levels. Therefore, despite improved total testosterone levels, they struggle to see the positive effects of treatment. This is because they still have low free testosterone due to high SHBG. And it may take several months for their SHBG to normalize, leading to more free testosterone and improved feelings of well-being.

Your lifestyle determines how quickly you see the effects of testosterone. If you eat a bad diet, drink a lot, and generally don't look after yourself, you may fail to see the positive effects of testosterone altogether until you address your lifestyle. Despite what some may think, **testosterone is not a panacea**.

For many men, one of the worst symptoms of low testosterone is the absence of libido, in addition to poor erection quality. Subsequently, one of the things men look forward to most with testosterone replacement therapy is increased libido. The good news is that libido and sexual function improve relatively quickly with treatment.

One meta-analysis reviewed studies on testosterone replacement therapy over a 35-year-period. They concluded that libido, sexual satisfaction, improved erections, and increased erection frequency can occur from three weeks up to 30 days. It's important to note that endothelial function (blood flow), or lack thereof, can be a major cause of erectile dysfunction. And poor blood flow can be the result of inflammation. Testosterone administration can improve inflammatory markers, including c-reactive protein (CRP) within three weeks. It can also promote the production of nitric oxide (necessary for blood flow to the penis) within four weeks.

Testosterone has a positive impact on your insulin sensitivity. Ultimately, the higher your insulin sensitivity, the better your health will be. High insulin sensitivity means your body is efficient at processing carbohydrates and requires less insulin to do so. Low insulin sensitivity on the other hand, or insulin resistance, means the body has to produce more insulin to metabolize glucose (i.e., carbohydrates). This leads to health problems such as high blood pressure and type 2 diabetes.

Furthermore, high levels of insulin and glucose (from insulin resistance) are toxic to the endothelium, resulting in inflammation, heart disease, and elevated oxidation.[254] Therefore, increasing your insulin sensitivity is in your best interests. Improvements in insulin sensitivity can be observed within just a week of undergoing testosterone replacement therapy. In addition, decreases in triglycerides may be noted after three months, extending all the way up to 12 months. Total cholesterol levels also decrease from between from four weeks up to the three-month mark.[255]

Another benefit many men look forward to on TRT is building lean muscle tissue. And who doesn't want to be bigger and stronger? One study administered 200 mg of testosterone enanthate every two weeks over the course of 36 months to men with low testosterone. They noted that significant increases in muscle tend to occur within

---

254    Osborn, *Get Serious.*

255    Farid Saad, Antonio Aversa, Andrea M Isidori, Livia Zafalon, Michael Zitzmann, and Louis Gooren, "Onset of effects of testosterone treatment and time span until maximum effects are achieved," *Eur J Endocrinol,* 2011 Nov; 165(5): 675–685. doi: 10.1530/EJE-11-0221.

the first 12 months.[256] And as we'll see in the chapter Building Your Body with Testosterone, your first year on TRT is crucial to building muscle mass.

In summary, the effects of testosterone don't occur suddenly; rather, they appear gradually over the course of several weeks or months. These changes can be subtle at first, but in time the change becomes noticeable.

## MONITORING YOUR TREATMENT

You should expect to have follow-up lab tests 6–8 weeks after you undergo treatment. This follow-up procedure is crucial because your physician will be able to see how your body responds to your treatment. Once again, how you feel in relation to your symptoms is the most important factor. Do you feel relief? Or do you still experience many of your symptoms?

If you still experience many of your symptoms after 6–8 weeks, that doesn't necessarily mean treatment doesn't work (as we'll see in a moment). We are all biochemically unique, which means not everyone will respond in the same manner to the same treatment.

It may take several iterations of your protocol and numerous lab tests until your physician understands what works best for you. As a result, you may need follow-up blood tests after your initial test. For example, you may start off injecting with 200 mg of testosterone a week. However, after blood work and consulting with your physician,

---

256    Stephanie T. Pagem John K. Amory, F. DuBois Bowman, Bradley D. Anawalt, Alvin M. Matsumoto, William J. Bremner, J. Lisa Tenover, "Exogenous Testosterone (T) Alone or with Finasteride Increases Physical Performance, Grip Strength, and Lean Body Mass in Older Men with Low Serum T," *The Journal of Clinical Endocrinology & Metabolism*, Volume 90, Issue 3, 1 March 2005: 1502–1510, https://doi.org/10.1210/jc.2004-1933.

you decide together that 175 mg a week would be a more appropriate dose. Because this is the dose where you feel your best.

After your initial 6–8 week follow-up, you should take another blood test approximately six months later to monitor how your body is responding. In most cases, this is a routine test because your doctor should already have a clear idea of what dose and injection frequency work best for you. After that, you should have another blood test on the year mark of your first year on TRT. Once again, this is a routine procedure to ensure that everything is okay. Then going forward, you should aim to have blood work done every 6–12 months.

## WHEN TESTOSTERONE DOESN'T WORK

Many men read rave reviews about TRT on the Internet. As a result, they have extremely high expectations for testosterone. Oftentimes, they expect testosterone to initiate dramatic changes within a few weeks. Again, this expectation is rooted in the instant gratification mindset that everything MUST happen immediately. So when results fail to materialize in the way they anticipated (i.e., rapid improvements in libido, mood, cognitive function, etc.), they become disillusioned and think testosterone "doesn't work."

However, to be clear—testosterone is not the problem. Men looking to testosterone for help need to start out with realistic expectations. Here are the key things to understand:

- Seeing changes with testosterone therapy takes time—up to several months in some cases. It takes time to get "dialed in" and properly adjusted to treatment. Unfortunately, nowadays patience is not a virtue, as everyone wants immediate results.

- Be on your guard against inappropriate treatment protocols. For example, your doctor prescribes TRT and you inject 200 mg of testosterone cypionate once every two weeks. You feel great after your initial injection, but 5–7 days later your blood testosterone levels begin to drop. As a result, you feel anxious, your energy declines, and your mood is affected.

Now you have to wait until the next injection. But worse still, you may have to go to your doctor's office to get it! These up and down fluctuations in blood testosterone levels are known as "peaks and valleys"—a side effect of a treatment protocol more suited to the Middle Ages. In this example, it's the antiquated treatment protocol that's the problem—not testosterone. That's why it is **imperative** to find the right doctor to treat you.

- According to Dr. Rob Kominiarek, MD, some men may feel a heightened sense of anxiety and nervousness after starting TRT—despite the fact TRT has been shown to improve feelings of anxiety in hypogonadal men. Increased anxiety after undergoing TRT is rare, but it can occur. This is thought to occur due to the suppression of LH, which is vital for the conversion of cholesterol into pregnenolone, as well as DHEA.[257] Research suggests that DHEA and pregnenolone have antidepressant and anxiolytic (i.e., anxiety-reducing) effects.[258] Therefore, this may explain why some men experience anxiety after undergoing TRT.

Dr. Kominiarek explains, "Pregnenolone, progesterone, allo-progesterone, allopregnenolone and allopregnanolone are

---

257   Aydogan U et al., "Increased frequency of anxiety, depression, quality of life and sexual life in young hypogonadotropic hypogonadal males and impacts of testosterone replacement therapy on these conditions," *Endocr J*, 2012, 59(12): 1099–105, epub 2012 Aug 31.

258   Rebecca K. Sripada, Ph.D., Robert C. Welsh, Ph.D., Christine E. Marx, M.D., Israel Liberzon, M.D., "The Neurosteroids Allopregnanolone and DHEA Modulate Resting-State Amygdala Connectivity," *Hum Brain Mapp*, 2014 Jul, 35(7): 3249–3261, published online 2013 Dec 2, doi: 10.1002/hbm.22399.

hormones that are responsible not only for short-term memory but also for cognition, mood, inflammation, mitochondrial function, and keeping us calm. When you take testosterone, you are altering brain chemistry. Many individuals, after the initiation of therapy, develop anxiety due to the loss of these hormones."[259]

## TESTOSTERONE, THE MAGIC BULLET?

Few things have the power to transform lives like testosterone. However, I want to make one thing crystal clear: **Testosterone is no magic bullet**. Guys think by virtue of taking testosterone all their problems will be solved and they will turn into Superman. But here's the thing— testosterone is the *catalyst* for change and not the change itself. Hormonal balance and testosterone are the foundation for positive change in your life. But if you do not build on that foundation with positive habits and actions, <u>it will do nothing for you.</u>

Testosterone is the DOING hormone, not the sitting around at home one. It will give you the motivation to go to the gym, more self-confidence in social situations, and energy to drive your career forward. But it's still up to you to lift weights, approach the girl, and take action in your life—testosterone won't do it for you.

---

259  Campbell, *The Testosterone Optimization Therapy Bible.*

# INTERVIEW WITH DR. KEITH NICHOLS

Dr. Keith Nichols is originally from Georgia and received his medical degree from the Medical College of Georgia in Augusta, Georgia. Following an internship at Spartanburg Regional Medical Center in Spartanburg, South Carolina, he completed his residency in Physical Medicine and Rehabilitation at the University of Louisville in Louisville, Kentucky.

He is board certified in Physical Medicine and Rehabilitation. He has served as a team physician for the Nashville Predators of the National Hockey league, a ringside physician for Strikeforce and the UFC, and has consulted in the care of many high school, college, and professional athletes. These include the Nashville Kats of the Arena Football League and the Tennessee Titans of the NFL.

**Daniel Kelly:** Dr. Nichols, why is hormone replacement therapy such an important topic, and why do you feel so passionate about it?

**Dr. Nichols:** That's an easy answer. It comes down to personal experience. I would not be where I am right now if I had not gone through the terrible symptoms of low testosterone. I don't know how accurately you can convey to someone just how bad that can be; the exhaustive fatigue, lack of mental clarity, irritability, and interruption to your sleep-wake cycle. Also, I hurt all over and didn't respond to any conventional medical treatments.

I lost the ability to exercise and if I did, I struggled to recover. I was just living a miserable existence, and I got to the point where I didn't want to do anything. So I went to my physician, and they tested me, and my total testosterone was 254 ng/dL (8.8 nmol/L). And, of course, according to the reference range, I was normal! So I went through everything that guys go through today. I was told I was just getting old and that was that. They even gave me a bunch of sleep aids that I almost became addicted to! And because I was tired all the time, I thought I might even have cancer. So they tested me for that and that came back negative. I couldn't take SSRIs, as they had too many side effects. It was really affecting my work, and I couldn't keep my eyes open in the afternoon.

I started doing research and realized my issue could be due to testosterone deficiency. So I got a prescription for a low-dose testosterone gel. However, I didn't get much of a response from it. Subsequently, I looked at other treatment options. At that time pellets were very popular, so I had them inserted. I actually started to feel much better, but you have a roller-coaster ride with pellets. You have to get one inserted every 3–4 months, and I didn't have enough body fat for them to insert it correctly. It was also expensive—$4,000 a year.

After my experience on pellets, I went onto injections once every two weeks then progressed to every other day injections. Eventually, I decided I didn't really like injecting all the time, so I experimented with a 20% compounded testosterone cream. I applied this to my chest and upper arm and got good results, but I had to use a lot. So I did more research, and with the help of Dr. Neal Rouzier, I decided to try a scrotal application for the testosterone cream. And, actually, the scrotum is the ideal place to apply a cream. The only reason you're told not to apply it there is because the gels contain alcohol that would burn your skin.

Every one of my patients who've used the scrotal application has done great. I don't receive phone calls about estrogen symptoms, and they're all very happy. Ultimately, through experimentation, I discovered the effectiveness of scrotal application. Nevertheless, my patients get a choice on whether they want to use injections or a cream. But once they try the scrotal application, they never go back. The good thing about the twice-daily application is that you don't get any peaks and troughs. You don't experience the dips you get when you have injections every two weeks or once a week, for example [because testosterone levels decline]. If you wanted to get the same effect of transdermal scrotal application with injectables, then you would have to do twice-daily injections. Nobody is going to do that.

**Daniel Kelly:** I've seen men who take creams and gels, yet they don't see much improvement of symptoms with them. As a result, they conclude TRT doesn't work. Why do gels and creams fail to work? Is it due to the application or the concentration of the solution?

**Dr. Nichols:** It can be both. If I compare taking transdermal creams when applied to any other body part [other than the scrotum] to daily injections, then I'll take injections. The reason most men don't get a response from creams and gels is because the concentration is not high enough. The highest concentration for a transdermal cream is 200 mg per gram. Whereas with an alcohol-based gel, like Androgel, it's 100 mg per gram. If you're going to use an alcohol-based application method, you're not going to get enough testosterone. In addition, you're probably not going to be able to apply enough to get a response, as it can be cost-prohibitive to use so much gel.

Essentially, with the transdermal scrotal application, you get all the benefits without the side effects. Although your levels can go up too much if you're not careful. When you use a scrotal application, your total testosterone can rise to 1500–2000 ng/dL (40–69 nmol/L) in the blink of an eye. You have to start off slow and see how it improves your symptoms. The typical dose for patients is 100 mg, so that's two clicks twice a day.

**Daniel Kelly:** How important is testosterone to the preventive medicine process?

**Dr. Nichols:** Testosterone affects every organ system. It protects the cardiovascular, neurological, musculoskeletal, and immune systems to name a few. The chronic diseases of aging are what cause problems as we grow older, and testosterone helps prevent that. A big killer for most people, at least in America, is an increase in visceral body fat. This increase in fat tissue releases inflammatory cytokines, which expose us to over 12 forms of cancer, including colorectal, breast, and prostate cancer. And not to mention diabetes and metabolic syndrome.

Testosterone protects against Alzheimer's, cardiovascular disease, cerebrovascular disease, hypertension, and diabetes. It decreases cholesterol and improves your lipid profile, it promotes healing—even in diabetics, increases lean muscle mass and libido, and reduces subcutaneous and visceral body fat. Ultimately, it increases the psychological well-being and health of the men who take it. Therefore, it's vital to maintain your hormones at an optimal level.

**Daniel Kelly:** Nowadays, physicians and patients alike get fixated on lab numbers. But what does an "optimal" level of testosterone actually mean?

**Dr. Nichols:** I treat based on symptom improvement. For me, an optimal level of testosterone is where someone with testosterone deficiency sees a dramatic improvement in their symptoms. "Optimal" is a level where you function at your best and you're healthy. Being optimal allows you to maintain your health by not becoming frail.

**Daniel Kelly:** Why are so many people still skeptical about testosterone?

**Dr. Nichols:** Pharmaceutical companies made a big marketing push with gels and creams, and mainstream medicine feels it's a fabricated disorder, made up by men. Similarly, the symptoms of testosterone deficiency can be related to many other disorders. Therefore, physicians may think a patient's issue is not necessarily low testosterone. They're also skeptical that testosterone deficiency exists in the presence of a "normal" testosterone value [on a lab test]. We've become a lab-centric (i.e., reliant on blood tests) versus a patient-centric medical society.

This parallels with how doctors used to treat thyroid deficiency. In the past, they would treat based on symptoms alone, but now it's all based on blood tests. For over a hundred years, they would treat based on symptoms alone. Then they would adjust the dosage until you got relief. Today, however, we've forgotten how to treat the patient and their symptoms. Instead, we treat numbers on a piece of paper.

Why do physicians treat numbers? You could say they're pressed for time, under pressure or whatever. But, honestly, it makes life easier to tick a box and follow a number. Doctors want everything nice and streamlined. And if they have to sit down with a patient for 20–30 minutes at a time, they might not make the income they want. For many family physicians, it's all about doing 6–10 minute consults and getting people through the door. They give out prescriptions quickly. Don't have a sex drive, or you're tired all the time? Great! Here's an antidepressant.

The reason I understand this so well is because I was one of those doctors. Everything was black and white. That's the way I was trained. Then you're around colleagues who do the same thing, so anyone who does different is "crazy." A typical scenario is this: The doctor draws your blood and the results tell him everything is "normal." Then the nurse calls to tell you your results are normal. Then you're at home thinking, *But why do I still feel like this and have all these symptoms? But the doctor says it's normal so it must be okay.* I see this all the time. Patients come in and say their doctor told them they're normal, but they feel terrible.

**Daniel Kelly:** How did you change your mentality from this black-and-white, lab-based doctor to one that treats patients based on symptoms?

**Dr. Nichols:** Because I went through **the misery of low testosterone**, and in many ways I was fortunate to experience it because now I know what patients go through. You cannot experience true empathy unless you've really been there. I myself went through a prostate cancer scare recently. For two weeks, my waking hours were filled with dread about cancer. It turns your world completely upside down. This gave me insight into patients who are diagnosed with cancer. Fortunately, the diagnosis turned out to be a false positive. And when it comes to low testosterone, you don't know what it's like until you have it. This whole experience made me see the dark side of medicine, which forced me to change.

**Daniel Kelly:** When we think of low testosterone, we assume you either produce enough testosterone or you don't. However, according to you, it's not just low testosterone that's the problem, but the actual cellular metabolism of testosterone as well. You call this "testosterone resistance." Can you elaborate on this?

**Dr. Nichols:** That's a great question, and I'm glad you asked. You'll be one of the first to talk about it in your book. The symptoms of testosterone deficiency can occur at multiple levels. We typically focus on things that are external to the cell (i.e., the production and level of testosterone in the blood). So we have primary and secondary hypogonadism, but you can also have symptoms of testosterone deficiency if you have decreased cellular tissue response. As we age, our organs don't work as well as they did when we were younger, so the cells don't respond as well. But what I'm really talking about is interference in the cellular metabolism of testosterone and defect in what's known as "signal transduction."

Signal transduction is a process that testosterone must go through to exert an effect. You can have symptoms of low testosterone if you're not producing enough of it. You can also have symptoms if too much free testosterone is bound up with sex hormone binding globulin (SHBG). But we currently don't have any way of measuring the cellular metabolism of testosterone. The testosterone has to enter the cell, diffuse through the cell membrane, and bind to the androgen receptor.

All men have different numbers of androgen receptors and different sensitivity to testosterone. So, the testosterone has to bind to the androgen receptor in the cell, and anything that blocks the binding of testosterone will result in symptoms of low testosterone. Once the testosterone is bound to the androgen receptor, it has to go into the nucleus of the cell, where it binds to the DNA. This process is known as *transcription*.

Anything that interferes with this process can also cause symptoms of low testosterone because testosterone's mechanism of action within the cell is being blocked. There are multiple levels at which testosterone can be affected, and this can occur even if blood levels of testosterone are normal outside the cell.

In my opinion, the reason this is happening is due to endocrine disrupting chemicals (EDCs). That is, any chemical that interferes with hormone action. Because we live in a toxic environment, all of us are exposed to these chemicals. They can block or bind to the androgen receptor and mimic the effect of estrogen. As a result, men get estrogenic symptoms (i.e., man boobs, love handles, etc.)

and women get breast cancer. In summary, we have interference with signal transduction, resulting in testosterone resistance.

Therefore, testosterone resistance can be the only answer for these guys who live a clean lifestyle yet still have the symptoms of low testosterone. As a young man, there is no reason you should have low testosterone other than due to the toxic environment. When I was younger, this didn't happen. The increase in low testosterone among young men correlates directly with the increase in production of EDCs in the last few decades. There are thousands of these chemicals in our environment, yet we only get to test for a handful of them. And I'm convinced EDCs are why you yourself went through low testosterone at 28.

# CHAPTER 12

# FINDING THE RIGHT DOCTOR

While it's true most of the medical establishment is stuck in the Dark Ages regarding testosterone replacement therapy, you can still find progressive doctors to treat you. For all the physicians out there that do not understand TRT, there are numerous smart, progressive physicians leading the way such as Dr. John Crisler, Dr. Merrill Matschke, and Dr. Keith Nichols. Guys often complain to me that they cannot find a doctor. But my response is always the same: If you truly need medical treatment, how badly do you want it? Because if you're really suffering, you'll do whatever it takes.

You'd better be prepared to travel for several hours or get on a plane to find the right doctor. This is the reality of the situation you face. However, if you're not willing to do that, I suggest you stop reading this book. I had to travel the length of the UK to obtain a prescription—a round trip that took over five hours. Was it worth it? You bet, because it completely changed the trajectory of my life, and I shudder to think how my life would have turned out otherwise.

So how do you find the right doctor? I believe getting a personal recommendation from an existing patient is the best route. If you know someone under the care of a TRT physician, and their treatment is going well and they feel great, that should be your first port of call.

The importance of finding the right doctor cannot be overstated. You cannot settle for a doctor simply because they prescribe testosterone therapy. It's a step up from not getting treatment; however, a poorly managed treatment protocol from an incompetent physician can prove as disastrous as low testosterone itself, as affirmed by Dr.

John Crisler: "TRT must be properly managed, and if it is not being administered by a physician who is knowledgeable in the field, these risks can be very serious … just like for every other medical therapy in existence."[260]

To obtain a prescription for testosterone replacement therapy, you must educate yourself and understand it way more than the average person—and in many cases better than your doctor. Without this knowledge, you may miss out on treatment altogether. Worse still, you run the risk of undergoing a haphazard treatment protocol because you don't know any better. Nevertheless, it's not only about avoiding substandard treatment protocols; you want to ensure you get an OPTIMAL treatment protocol.

The whole point of undergoing TRT is to live an **exceptional quality of life**. Why go to all the trouble to just feel okay? Possessing this knowledge allows you to effectively screen out AVERAGE and incompetent doctors because the decision to undergo TRT will be one of the biggest decisions you ever make—but also one of the best.

While you are committed to a lifelong treatment and all it entails, both psychologically and financially, you are simultaneously committed to GREAT health. In this chapter we look at the steps you need to take to find the right doctor. Although with the odds so stacked against them, it's any wonder young men can get a prescription for testosterone at all.

Time and again, patients meekly accept a doctor's verdict simply because they are in a position of authority. Extensive training and years of medical school make doctors experts in medicine. But that does not mean they are experts in ALL fields of medicine—*especially* TRT. The days of blindly following the doctor's advice are over. Take

---

260   Dr. John Crisler, *Testosterone Replacement Therapy: A Recipe for Success* (Amazon Digital Services, 2015).

control of your own destiny with the information contained in this chapter.

## 12 QUESTIONS FOR YOUR TRT DOCTOR

Given most doctors don't know the first thing about TRT, how do you know if you can trust them? To be clear, you don't have to interview hundreds of doctors or spend hours reading endocrinology textbooks to see if a doctor is right for you. By asking some basic questions, you can build up a clear picture of their approach to hormone therapy. The following are questions you should ask your TRT physician.

### 1) What testosterone administration protocol do they prefer—injection, creams, or other?

Intramuscular injections, and in some cases subcutaneous injection, are preferred methods of treatment. As seen in the previous chapter, when used properly, a case for creams can also be made. However, if your doctor proposes a worthless treatment such as pellets or lozenges, seek an alternative.

### 2) Do they allow you to have input on the kind of treatment you want?

If a doctor is open to input from you on your treatment, that's the sign of a great doctor. Incompetent doctors who think they know everything dictate the terms; they're closed to input from patients on how their treatment should look.

### 3) What dosage protocol do they advise and how often?

Your doctor should have a good understanding of pharmacokinetics (i.e., the half-life of a drug) and their effect on blood testosterone levels. Ideally, they should ask you to inject at a MINIMUM of once a week. If your TRT doctor advises you to inject once every couple of weeks, this is a telltale sign of a doctor living in the Dark Ages, and you must find another.

## 4) How many patients have they treated for hypogonadism?

Some doctors may prescribe testosterone but may not necessarily specialize in hormone optimization. Therefore, it's a good idea to understand how many men they've actually treated for hypogonadism. Although it must be stressed—it's not necessarily how many people they've treated, but their overall philosophy regarding hormone optimization that is important.

## 5) Do they have experience treating young men?

Some doctors will not treat younger patients because of potential risks to fertility and fear of being sued (mostly in the US). Some even think young men don't need TRT, regardless of their situation. Do they offer testosterone, or do they prefer to prescribe hCG or Clomid? If so, why?

## 6) Do they require you to take an AI with your treatment? If so, why?

Some doctors prescribe estrogen control methods when patients exhibit high estrogen symptoms, and even then, they do so reluctantly. Other physicians prescribe anti-estrogens from the outset. In either case, you must understand their rationale for it. As discussed in the previous chapter, in an ideal scenario, you should aim to avoid AIs altogether.

## 7) Do they provide other therapies that can complement testosterone replacement?

Do they offer ancillary medications that complement your treatment and improve health and well-being?

## 8) Do they allow you to self-inject?

If you go the injection route, you want to become self-reliant. You do not want to visit the doctor's office every week to get an injection. You'll accumulate unnecessary bills and waste time traveling for a procedure that takes 20 seconds at home.

## 9) How often do you have to go see them?

After you've received your prescription and your protocol is dialed in, you should have reviews and blood work every 6–12 months. Anything more than this and I would be suspicious of the doctor's motives.

## 10) Do they share blood work results with you?

Your doctor should be open to sharing your blood work with you. After all, it is your health! You must take responsibility for your own health and ask for a copy of your blood work. If they are unwilling to share your medical information with you, you must question their motives. You should not be kept in the dark about any aspect of treatment and not accept any doctor-knows-best behavior.

## 11) What is the set-up fee and ongoing cost of labs and drugs?

A doctor's practice may seem very attractive due to low set-up fees. But once you go ahead, you may get hit by hidden ongoing costs. Make sure the practice is transparent with you and you understand all costs upfront.

## 12) Are they in good physical health themselves and/or do they take testosterone?

Personally, I find that if a doctor is out of shape and in bad health themselves, I cannot take them seriously. How can you preach about health when yours is a mess? Furthermore, your doctor doesn't HAVE to take testosterone because there may not be a medical need for it. But if he does take it, that's a good sign. It means he practices what he preaches. Indeed, the leading doctors I have mentioned in this book—Dr. John Crisler, Dr. Keith Nichols, and Dr. Merrill Matschke—are all on TRT themselves and are in fantastic shape. It stands to reason that if a doctor takes good care of himself, he will take care of his patients.

## THE DANGERS OF POLYPHARMACY

*Polypharmacy* is the use of multiple medications to treat one or more conditions—a phenomenon typically seen in elderly patients with multiple chronic illnesses.[261] However, this practice is no longer confined to the elderly; it has filtered down to the general population.

Polypharmacy occurs frequently in modern medicine because treatment is so compartmentalized. For example, the endocrinologist treats a patient for one condition, the neurologist for another, and so on. As a result, patients end up with a laundry list of medications and different treatment protocols that often contradict each other. However, it's not the medical system alone that is to blame—most patients blindly accept a doctor's diagnosis without thinking for themselves. They would prefer to pop pills to cure themselves instead of fixing the root cause.

---

261   Nashwa Masnoon Sepehr Shakib, Lisa Kalisch-Ellett, and Gillian E. Caughey, "What is polypharmacy? A systematic review of definitions," *BMC Geriatr*, 2017, 17: 230, published online 2017 Oct 10, doi: 10.1186/s12877-017-0621-2.

I've seen this attitude toward polypharmacy firsthand in patients who undergo TRT. It's as though the floodgates open once they've committed themselves to treatment. Much like being in a candy store, they want to take as many drugs as possible under the guise of "optimizing" their health. <u>But taking more drugs doesn't necessarily equate to better results.</u>

People have become so desensitized to the idea of taking drugs that using multiple medications is now like brushing your teeth. This is due to limited time and resources and the reality that doctors are more willing to prescribe multiple medications. But what people need to realize is that more drugs mean more side effects, management, and cost. Indeed, some drugs can actually counteract the effects of others. Just as I say to my coaching clients that "You can't out-train a bad diet"—nor can more drugs make up for a poor lifestyle.

If you must take multiple medications, take one at a time. For instance, if you take hCG alongside testosterone, don't take them both at the same time from the beginning. Instead, the idea is to get adjusted on one medication first—for example, take testosterone, then introduce the other one several weeks or even months later, only AFTER symptoms and blood work have been assessed. If you don't do this, you won't know how each medication affects your body, and as a result, your physician won't know how to monitor and adjust your treatment properly. This is a crucial step in getting your treatment right.

# INTERVIEW WITH DR. MERRILL MATSCHKE

One of the leading figures and torchbearers in hormone optimization is Dr. Merrill Matschke. He is a Board Certified urologist who is fellowship trained in Male Reproductive Medicine and Surgery. I have a lot of respect for Dr. Matschke, and I wanted to interview him here for a number of reasons. First, because he is almost unparalleled in his knowledge of hormone optimization and has extensive practical experience in treatment. As a result, he treats patients based on what actually works, as opposed to relying on arbitrary recommendations from an endocrinology textbook.

Dr. Matschke is himself a patient of testosterone replacement therapy, while living and breathing a lifestyle conducive to good health—talk about practicing what you preach! Finally, I admire the fact Dr. Matschke has had the courage to speak out against demonization and malpractice of testosterone therapy, knowing it might cost him opportunities or set him up to be ostracized. We need more voices like Dr. Matschke's to give weight and credibility to the positive message that is hormone optimization.

**Daniel Kelly:** Dr. Matschke, why do you think so many physicians today are hesitant to treat young men?

**Dr. Matschke:** This is most likely due to the gross misinformation and pervasive lack of information available in standard medical teaching today regarding hypogonadism. The tendency amongst physicians is to avoid what you don't understand. Furthermore, when you combine an absent fund of knowledge with a scenario involving younger patients, there is more at risk for the poorly trained physician. The natural inclination of virtually all providers is to brush off, avoid, or even chastise a younger man with suboptimal testosterone. This is the sad reality of today's mass-market medical system.

Physicians, many of whom began their journey into medicine with an altruistic core, are wrung out, burnt out, and oftentimes cynical. Instead of listening to the concerns of younger men and maintaining an up-to-date knowledge base regarding endocrine disruption and its catastrophic significance, the typical provider falls back to historical myths that testosterone is dangerous, only abused, and causes fertility problems.

**Daniel Kelly:** In the past you've commented on the population level decline of testosterone. In your experience, how prevalent is low testosterone among young men, and how often do you see them in your own practice?

**Dr. Matschke:** This is a fascinating situation. It is undoubtedly at an all-time high, but the complicating factor is the continuing controversy of defining "low testosterone." So the answer requires a bit of an explanation. In the United States, for example, current insurance-based medical practice requires total testosterone to be below 300 ng/dL (10.4 nmol/L) for a diagnosis of hypogonadism to be established. Unfortunately, this criterion is wholly inadequate to define what is a complex clinical syndrome. Nevertheless, if you apply this archaic scheme to my prior practice in male reproductive medicine, my experience was at least 50% of younger men suffered from a total T less than 300 ng/dL.

To be fair, there is selection bias by applying this to my practice because I saw a high percentage of men in couples having difficulties achieving pregnancy. Understand, however, that there was only a male factor to their infertility in about <u>30% of cases</u>. Thus, this still represents an obvious signal for a higher than previously reported prevalence of hypogonadism in younger men.

Now, if we recognize that younger men should have the highest levels of testosterone—namely in the 700–1,100 ng/dL range (24.3– 38 nmol/L)—then the story is much more staggering. Testosterone is known to be at its highest in younger men. It peaks in the late teens through to the late twenties and then begins to fall about age 30. Therefore, if I apply this more appropriate, clinically based, rationale, I would put the prevalence in the neighborhood of 80%. I have been noting this for the past 10+ years and trying to convey its significance, only to fall on deaf ears. At a time in a man's life when his testosterone should be at its peak, the vast majority of those young men have testosterone levels in the lower half to lower quartile range (i.e., bottom end of the reference range). It is really astounding, but more troubling is the utter lack of urgency displayed by our modern medical system.

**Daniel Kelly:** Many young men are confused about which treatment is right for them. In what instances is it advised for a young man to take exogenous testosterone versus Clomid or hCG, for example?

**Dr. Matschke:** This is where I put my Andrologist hat on. If a young man has suboptimal testosterone and any future interest in fathering children, he must have a high-quality semen analysis performed and reviewed by a qualified provider. The testes have two primary outputs: sperm and testosterone. So if a young man is deficient in testosterone, it's necessary for him to evaluate the status of his spermatogenesis (sperm production) as well.

All younger men also MUST have their gonadotropins (LH and FSH) pre-evaluated, as this will differentiate between primary versus secondary testis failure. If a young man shows evidence of low LH (less so low FSH), he may very well be best served by hCG or Clomid. These represent more of modality of "T support," as they increase production of endogenous testosterone. As a side benefit, hCG or clomiphene can also improve the quality of semen parameters. In fact, I often use these approaches in younger men who have low sperm counts and/or quality and are trying to conceive.

However, some men may not get the improvement in symptoms they desire with hCG or clomiphene. In these individuals, exogenous testosterone may be considered, albeit only after a thorough discussion regarding potential negative impacts on future fertility potential. If these men elect to use exogenous testosterone, it is best to co-administer with either hCG or clomiphene at modified doses to protect and maintain spermatogenesis. While not mandatory, this approach provides the best protection against reduction of endogenous testis function. Even when co-administration with hCG or clomiphene is elected, I strongly advise periodic follow-up semen analyses to ensure that sperm production isn't impacted. The earliest these should be done is 3–4 months after starting the therapy.

Another group of young men that would have to consider exogenous testosterone use would be those that suffer from primary testis failure, as neither hCG nor clomiphene would be effective for increasing endogenous T. These men most often will have associated severe defects in sperm production, so they already have a diminished fertility potential. At the very least, these individuals should entertain cryopreservation of sperm for future advanced reproductive techniques (IVF or insemination) prior to initiating therapy. Ideally, these men should be evaluated and counseled by a subspecialist in male infertility.

**Daniel Kelly:** Fertility is a major concern for any young men undergoing TRT. Although, many who undergo treatment are still not ready for children. Should they maintain their fertility from the beginning by using hCG alongside testosterone, or can they restore fertility later on when they are ready to father children?

**Dr. Matschke:** Ideally, I advise co-administration of hCG or clomiphene with TRT in young men wishing to optimally maintain their future fertility potential. This will do everything possible to prevent a negative impact on sperm production. Those who choose to use *appropriate* TRT alone will, on average, suppress their sperm production to infertile levels (less than 1 million sperm) within 3.5 months of starting TRT. The good news is that 90% of men will recover their prior level of sperm production within 12 months of stopping *appropriate* TRT if they want to attempt having children. By two full years of being off exogenous testosterone, 99% of men will have returned to their pre-TRT sperm production levels.

Additionally, there are approaches that can "jump-start" the return of sperm production after TRT. This is NOT to say that all young men using any androgenic steroids (synthetics and supraphysiologic doses) will regain normal sperm production at any time period. Using inappropriate high doses and/or synthetic anabolics can potentially have a more permanent negative impact on sperm production. So understanding that fertility can be affected is important, but we absolutely can protect and preserve future fertility when responsibly achieving optimal testosterone levels.

**Daniel Kelly:** Given they are often in the early stages of their careers, do you think young men see the cost of hormone optimization as a big obstacle?

**Dr. Matschke:** I do not. The average monthly cost of injectable testosterone and supplies is $30–$40. That's literally just barely more than one dollar a day. There are cash-only providers that will manage this for about $1,000 per year. This represents a miniscule investment in long-term health. If one can get doctor visits covered by insurance (and can find an enlightened/capable insurance-based provider) then, in theory, it could even be less expensive for ongoing monitoring.

**Daniel Kelly:** Finally, why is there such a lack of knowledge from a physician and patient standpoint about the importance of testosterone to men's health? Is the lack of awareness down to ignorance alone or a failure in the medical and mainstream education system?

**Dr. Matschke:** I see this as a massive failure of our medical education system. There is a complete lack of adequate time spent on the systemic impacts of testosterone on human physiology. Not only is there a lack of time spent, there is an even deeper lack of educational material available. Today, this is an education that can only obtained by those with the intellectual curiosity to seek it out. Virtually nowhere is there relevant information regarding the importance of testosterone in cardiometabolic risk, endothelial dysfunction, insulin signaling, mental health, and the list goes on. Instead, teaching still focuses on outdated, inaccurate concepts such as testosterone being implicated in increased cardiovascular risk and prostate cancer.

Frankly, it is mainstream medical malpractice. We are slowly beginning to see some cracks in the mainstream wall of resistance, but it is taking much too long given the overwhelming amount of ironclad data/science supporting the role of testosterone in health and wellness. Thankfully, there exists a growing movement of preventive medicine that embraces the health-promoting aspects of optimal testosterone levels. In addition, there is a focused, grassroots phenomenon educating the public on the importance of testosterone as it relates to optimal living.

# CHAPTER 13

# BUILDING YOUR BODY WITH TESTOSTERONE

One of the incredible benefits of achieving optimal testosterone levels, whether with exogenous testosterone or through raising your natural levels, is the ability to gain lean muscle mass. And let's be clear, there is NOTHING wrong with gaining muscle, although society wants to make you feel bad for doing so, and would prefer you to be a weakling. When I discuss testosterone with men in the context of gaining muscle, I often hear, "I want to gain muscle, but I don't want to get too big!" At this point, I know they have little to no training experience. Gaining muscle is not a cakewalk—whether with testosterone or not. Not only do you have to be ruthless with your diet and training but also doggedly persistent.

It makes me laugh because most men don't know what it takes. They think by virtue of taking testosterone they will turn into the Hulk—if only it were that simple! Sorry, gentlemen, but testosterone doesn't provide a shortcut to muscle utopia. **You still have to work your ass off and pay your dues.** But if you're intelligent and make the right moves, you can expect to put on a decent amount of muscle. As the saying goes, "Build it and they will come."

It's almost as though men today have a guilt complex about building muscle—as if they should be ashamed of it. But please tell me, what's shameful about looking and feeling fantastic? Nothing. When guys feel ashamed in this manner, it's because they're are afraid to be men. Strength and power are at the core of your essence as a man. Nowadays, though, if you're physically strong you're an outlier. Some men may claim they don't want to be physically impressive, but deep down almost every man secretly wants to be—he's just been conditioned by society to pretend otherwise.

I want to give you permission right now to feel ZERO shame in your pursuit of realizing your full potential as a man—to build muscle and become stronger. Men were not destined to be weak. Stronger men make better fathers, husbands, and brothers, and they are more functional members of society. Indeed, we would be better off if more men invested in their physical and mental strength. **And despite what some say, no one respects a weak man.**

## HOW TO TRAIN AND GAIN MUSCLE

The training principles outlined in this chapter apply whether you are on testosterone replacement therapy or looking to raise your testosterone naturally. Nevertheless, if you do undergo testosterone replacement therapy, you will find your training capacity will significantly improve. You will be able tolerate more punishment than the average trainee. This also means you'll need less time off from training, which ultimately equates to more strength and muscle.

When I was a natural trainee, I could train for five to six weeks straight without rest. After that, I would need to take an entire week off resistance training to recover. Since I began testosterone, I can for go months on end without needing a break. Although training in this manner is not made possible by testosterone alone. There are a few principles you need to abide by to train for sustained periods and consistently get results.

Above all, you must understand your own body and how it responds to certain types of training. In addition, you need to know what type of foods work best for you and what type of diet supports your level of training. Does a low-carbohydrate approach work well for you? Or does your body tolerate higher amount of carbohydrates? How much rest do you need to be able to recover fully? Is three days a week in the gym enough for you, or do you need to do more?

At the ancient Greek site of Delphi, there is a famous inscription that reads, "Know thyself." This saying is as true for you as it was for battle-hardened Spartan warriors. Reading books on diet and training and watching YouTube videos are all great. But there are no shortcuts here, and you must experiment to discover <u>what works best for you</u>.

There are pros and cons to every type of training method and diet. That's why it's key to try different approaches and, in particular, to see what you enjoy. Because if you enjoy something, you're more likely to stick with it and achieve lasting results.

On another note, I often see guys go to the gym and try to train all-out intensity every time. However, the human body simply cannot support that level of training. Nor do you have to train 100% of your capacity every time to get results. This approach leads to burnout.

Make the decision now to accept you won't have a stellar workout every time you set foot in the gym. Of course, when you go to the gym, give it your all. Sometimes you will have exceptional workouts where you feel like an uncaged lion. And sometimes it will be completely flat. But the main thing is that you show up week in, week out. Keep showing up and your results will be assured. **Consistency always wins out.**

## THE BEAST MODE MINDSET

If you want results from your training, you must adopt the mindset of ALL OR NOTHING. This is what I call the "Beast Mode Mindset." Too often I see guys in the gym who are half-hearted in their efforts, and they train aimlessly without any real purpose. When you enter the gym, you must become like a warrior ready to do battle with the weights. If this idea is too extreme for you, the truth is you aren't willing to do what it takes to achieve extreme results.

You must become ruthlessly focused in your approach. Get rid of distractions and leave your phone in the locker. If you listen to music while you train, put your device in airplane mode. Also, there's no need to look at social media or take a phone call while you train (unbelievably, this does happen). Do you think Arnold Schwarzenegger or Jay Cutler would have built champion physiques if they constantly checked their Facebook status during workouts? Of course not! Their single-minded focus was the key to their success.

Nevertheless, there is a caveat with this mindset. There is a *firm distinction* between pushing your body beyond your perceived limits and completely destroying your body so you cannot train for days. The first way is smart, the second is dumb and counterproductive, leading to burnout. As the great Mike Mentzer said, "Any exercise carried on beyond the least amount required to stimulate an optimal increase is not merely a waste of effort, it is actually highly counterproductive … [when you train] you are utilizing biochemical resources that must be replaced, and **the more you use the more that must be replaced**."[262]

There will be times when you train and feel weak, and you can't lift half of what you normally can. If this happens on more than one exercise, you should call it a wrap at the gym for the day or do some light cardio. Perhaps you're stressed, overtrained, sick, etc. Whatever it is, it's a sign that your body needs a rest, and there's no shame in that. Actually, it's an intelligent response. You must pick your battles; running yourself into the ground benefits no one. Listen to your body. You can't be a beast if you're always beaten down.

262   Mike Mentzer and John Little, *High Intensity Training the Mike Mentzer Way* (McGraw-Hill Education, 2003).

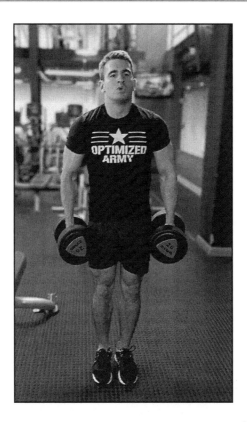

## THE MIND-MUSCLE CONNECTION

During exercise, your brain sends signals to your muscle fibers to contract. The more you can improve this neurological connection between your brain and muscles, the more muscle fibers you can recruit when you perform an exercise. More muscle fiber recruitment will result in better muscle contractions, better workouts, and more muscle growth. In bodybuilding circles, this is known as the *mind-muscle connection*, and science is now starting to catch up.

One study of 18 resistance-trained men looked at the importance of the mind-muscle connection during resistance training. The researchers wanted to see if focusing on specific muscle fibers increases their activation. Subjects performed three types of bench press: a regular bench press and two others that focused specifically on pectoral and triceps activation. Exercises were done at intensities of 20%, 40%, 60%, and 80% of subjects' one rep max (1RM). The researchers found that resistance-trained individuals can increase muscle fiber activation by actively focusing on the muscle involved, thereby substantiating the mind-muscle connection. Although it appears this is only possible at a threshold of between 60–80% of 1RM. [263] [264]

How do you develop the mind-muscle connection? There are many ways to do it. For example, when lifting, most guys just focus on lifting the weight up. But in reality, you should use just as much effort to lower a weight. Don't let gravity take over, aim to actively lower it and feel your muscles as you do it.

In addition, every time you flex your muscle at the top of a movement, for example at the top of a bicep curl, aim to squeeze the target muscle as much as possible. As former Mr. Olympia Lee Haney said, "Squeeze it like it owes you money!" This process drives blood into the muscle, thereby forcing the buildup of metabolic waste products, which help contribute to the repair and growth of muscle tissue.

Many of us have lost connection with our own bodies, due to sedentary and technology-centered lives. We no longer identify with our bodies; it's almost as if it's simply a vessel for the mind. This is also accentuated by Western culture that places emphasis on left-brain thinking.

---

263    Calatayud J, Vinstrup, Jakobsen MD, Sundstrup E, Brandt M, Jay K, Colado JC, Andersen LL, "Importance of mind-muscle connection during progressive resistance training," *Eur J Appl Physiol*, 2016 Mar, 116(3): 527–33, doi: 10.1007/s00421-015-3305-7.

264    For further study, see Calatayud J, Vinstrup J, Jakobsen MD, Sundstrup E, Colado JC, Andersen LL, "Mind-muscle connection training principle: influence of muscle strength and training experience during a pushing movement," *Eur J Appl Physiol*, 2017 Jul, 117(7): 1445--1452, doi: 10.1007/s00421-017-3637-6.

We spend most of our day stuck in our own head. So if you sit at a desk all day, there's a strong chance your motor neural pathways, particularly in your shoulders and upper back, are dormant or under-developed. You will have a poor mind-muscle connection that is exacerbated by poor posture from sitting at a keyboard. This can lead to nagging issues like shoulder impingement and elbow tendinitis.

If you are uncoordinated, a good way to develop a deeper connection with your body is to take up an activity that requires muscular coordination. Examples include rock climbing, dancing, or a team sport. I myself noticed improved muscular coordination after taking up dancing lessons. Before this, I struggled to feel and move many of the muscles in my body, particularly in my shoulders and upper back. But now I can do it with ease.

You can also use the power of visualization to improve the mind-muscle connection. Science tells us the brain doesn't know the difference between your imagination and perceived reality. Use this to your advantage. To use visualization in your workouts, start by doing your warm-up sets. Once you're warmed up, visualize the reps before every set you do. See yourself lift the weight, but also feel what it's like when your muscles contract and you lift the weight. If it's a weight you've never done before, see yourself lifting it effortlessly.

And sometime during the workout, take the time to visualize yourself with your ideal physique. Notice how it feels to be that person and have that kind of physique. Through this visualization process, you reprogram your subconscious mind. And eventually, the physique you visualize becomes your reality. Elite-level athletes use visualization all the time to achieve their goals, so why can't you?

## WORKING OUT YOUR EGO, AND THE IMPORTANCE OF PROPER FORM

Most understand the importance of using good form, but few take the time to actually do it. Most guys prefer to pile the weight on the bar in a misguided attempt to be "strong." But inevitably the weight ends up being too much, and they struggle to execute the exercise properly. This results in half-squats and deadlifts with a hunched back. This is what I call, "Working out your ego" because when you use too much weight, only your ego gets a workout.

Training with proper form isn't only for the anal-retentive—it serves a real purpose. Using proper form allows you to perform an exercise in a safe manner, thereby avoiding injury (CrossFit anyone?). When you're young with the world at your feet, you feel invincible. But stupid training practices will come back to haunt you. I know guys in their 50s who learned this lesson the hard way because they never took the time to manage their ego. In your 50s, a bicep tear or a sprained ankle may mean months out of the gym. Not only can you not train, but your quality of life is severely affected. Learn this lesson early on: When you go to the gym, leave your ego at the door.

Ego isn't all bad—it's what drives you to develop your physique in the first place. There is **nothing wrong** with wanting to look good naked. It makes you feel more attractive and confident. And only losers who are ashamed of their bodies will say otherwise. Nonetheless, there is a stark difference between channeling your ego positively versus allowing it to control you. I will have more to say on the subject of ego in the Balance and Spirituality chapter.

## CARVING THE DIAMOND

A common theme I see with guys in the gym is they try to do too much too soon. When it comes to building a quality physique, patience is a virtue. Sometimes guys jump headlong into training with enthusiasm, trying to train as much as possible. Then they become disillusioned when things don't happen quickly. Once again, this is because they're impatient and their expectations have no basis in reality. **One of the best things you can do for your fitness and life in general is learn to be more patient.**

Every time you go to the gym, aim to get a little bit better—even if it's just two pounds extra on the bar or a few more reps. Whatever it is, over time this compounds into <u>substantial progress</u>. I call this, "Carving the diamond." You need to view building your physique as a lifelong project. Consider how Michelangelo or Leonardo da Vinci viewed their paintings. Do you think they rushed so they could complete them sooner? Of course not; they understood a true masterpiece takes time.

Many young men suffer from a negative body image. No matter what they do, they can't feel confident about their bodies. But understand that you are not powerless. In fact, if there's one thing you have control over in your life—it's your body. If you can get off your ass and get to the gym, you can change your body and change your life. Your situation is never hopeless, but it is if you *choose* it to be. You must let go of comparing yourself to others, because **the only person you are ever in competition with is yourself.** The moment you start to compare your progress to others is the moment you lose focus. The success of others can be a motivational tool to push yourself, but beating yourself up about your perceived lack of progress will not serve you.

## HOW MUCH MUSCLE CAN YOU GAIN WITH TESTOSTERONE?

Your first year on testosterone replacement therapy is a great opportunity to gain a decent amount of muscle mass. This is because your androgen receptors become saturated with testosterone, perhaps for the first time if you've been suffering from chronic low testosterone, and subsequently up-regulate. Therefore, in your first year on testosterone therapy, if you train hard and eat right, you can expect to gain 5–10 lbs—and possibly more. I've heard stories of guys gaining up to 20 lbs in their first year, although these cases tend to be outliers.

The exact amount of muscle you gain will depend on a variety of factors, including genetics, training, recovery, diet, and lifestyle factors such as stress. I want to emphasize this is a once-in-a-lifetime opportunity. This is not to say you cannot continue to build muscle beyond your first year on testosterone, you just won't get the dramatic muscle growth that is possible in your first year.

And if you're new to lifting weights altogether, you're going to gain muscle no matter what. This is a result of the "rookie effect." The sudden stress placed on the body causes you to gain muscle in rapid succession. But even if you are an advanced trainee like I was, you can still expect to gain appreciable muscle mass, provided you train smart and eat right.

# CHAPTER 14

# LEADING A LIFE OF DISCIPLINE

Discipline has become a hot topic in recent times, and every year countless books are published on the subject. But leading a disciplined life is nothing new. Humans have long recognized the importance and rewards of a disciplined life. The word *discipline* itself means different things to different people, and this is reflected in the myriad definitions found in the dictionary. The one I like most is from *The Oxford Dictionary*: "A system of rules of conduct."[265] Essentially, that's all it is: Training your mind and body to behave a certain way. Being disciplined means you live consciously instead of unconsciously acquiring habits that thwart your progress. You consciously choose desired behaviors to achieve *specific* outcomes. And, eventually, these desired behaviors become habits.

In most cases, the only thing standing between us and our goal is ourselves. We get in our own way when we allow fear and doubt to dominate our thinking. With the right mindset, anyone can use discipline to achieve their goals and lead a more rewarding life.

One of the reasons I included this chapter is because discipline is misunderstood and is a virtue sorely lacking in many young men's lives. They drift aimlessly from one shiny object to another, trying whatever takes their fancy. They abandon things easily because they lack the staying power required to achieve anything.

Instant gratification from smartphones and video games has lured them into believing immediate results are the norm. When this

---

265   *Oxford Living Dicrionaries*, s.v., "Discipline," accessed January 9, 2019, https://en.oxforddictionaries.com/definition/discipline.

doesn't happen, they become disillusioned and lost, and it is discipline that will help them find their way.

I know you care deeply about your health, but I want to stress that without discipline, you will always be at the mercy of the whims of the mind and body. **Great health does not come without great discipline.**

## DEVELOP DISCIPLINE THROUGH RESISTANCE TRAINING

How do you incorporate discipline into your life? Indeed, the idea of becoming disciplined may seem so foreign to you that it becomes overwhelming. So you procrastinate and fail to take action altogether. <u>Understand that discipline must form the backbone of any meaningful change.</u>

Oftentimes, when people attempt to make big changes, they take on too much in a small space of time. As a result, they crash and burn. Imagine a guy who decides he wants to lose weight and do it quickly. He's been overweight for years, and he's tired of it. He may have even had periodic success losing weight after going on a crash diet—only for the weight to return with a vengeance a few months later. This is because he didn't develop the necessary discipline and address the habits that got him overweight in the first place.

Nowadays, you can find a plethora of books and blog posts that wax lyrical about all sorts of hacks and techniques you can use to become more disciplined. From waking up at 5 a.m., to taking cold showers, to doing yoga and breathing exercises. And don't get me wrong, these are all great things. However, there's an underlying assumption that if you follow these techniques to the letter, you too will develop the discipline of a Navy SEAL. Now, these things may work well for A-list celebrities and CEOs, but it doesn't mean they will work for you.

These hacks and tricks to build discipline place too much emphasis on external habits. Instead, focus on developing your character, on becoming a disciplined individual. Because, ultimately, discipline is not just a bunch of techniques—it's a mindset. If you don't have the correct mindset, it doesn't matter what technique you use.

*Excellence is an art won by training and habituation. We do not act rightly because we have virtue or excellence, but we rather have those because we have acted rightly. We are what we repeatedly do. Excellence, then, is not an act but a habit. —Aristotle*

The seeds of discipline are sown through small daily acts, and resistance training forms the backbone of a disciplined life. In the traditional sense, resistance training means using a form of resistance (i.e., weights or your own body weight to train your muscles). However, I want you to view resistance training as not only training for the body, but training for the mind too.

In his excellent book *Do the Work*, author Steven Pressfield says we all have innate resistance that sabotages us at every turn. This resistance prevents you from getting up in the morning, from writing a book, or even starting a business. Pressfield says resistance shows up with "any act that rejects immediate gratification in favor of long-term growth, health, or integrity."[266]

He goes on to say resistance will always be there, but when you kick its ass regularly, your mind believes in your ability to overcome

266    Steven Pressfield, Do the Work (The Domino Project/Black Irish Entertainment, 2014).

it. This is how you smash limiting beliefs—not by meditating or thinking about them, but by taking action *in spite* of them.

So how do you kick resistance's ass? In contrast to others, I don't believe in prescribing a bunch of techniques to develop discipline— you have enough of those already. Instead, I want you to see discipline as a mental muscle you develop alongside the physical muscles you develop in the gym.

Consider this: Every time you perform an exercise and grind out that last rep, even when it's hard and everything inside you tells you to stop, you develop your discipline muscle. Every time you go to the gym and maintain strict form on every exercise, even though your training partner uses more weight and your ego tells you that you can lift more, you develop your discipline muscle. Every time you go to the gym after work and pound the weights, even though you had a rough day and you're tired as shit, you develop your discipline muscle. Every time you train, even though your buddies are going out to get drunk, you develop your discipline muscle. When you go to the gym anyway, even though the gains are slow and it sometimes feels it's not working, you develop your discipline muscle. This is why I see the gym as a training ground for the mind as much as the body.

Once you make a conscious effort to train your mind in this manner, you begin to see discipline in everything you do. When you reach this point, discipline will become your identity, as opposed to something other people do. Even if you are a seasoned trainee, I urge you to take this approach to training, and your results will improve even more.

"Resistance training" in this sense can also be accomplished through martial arts. Getting punched in the face or tapped out on the mat is a humbling experience and a powerful way to train your mind. So is climbing a mountain; the act of putting one foot in front of the other and moving for hours in end, even when ever fiber in your body tells you to stop, is another powerful experience that will develop discipline.

Regardless of the physical activity you do choose, make sure it challenges you. The mind will always make up excuses not to do something and will only change its viewpoint when it's forced. Nevertheless, if you are reading this book and care about your health, lifting weights should become the cornerstone of your lifestyle. There are few things that don't benefit from increased strength.

The mind is whimsical by nature. It doesn't want to change and must be disciplined. Otherwise it will revert to its familiar, comfortable (i.e., undisciplined) ways. The discipline created through resistance training carries over to the rest of your life.

Over time your mind automatically disciplines itself, and you no longer have to worry about overcoming temptation. Offered a piece of cake at the office? No thanks. Fasting until 4p.m.? Easy. Doing 30 minutes of cardio? Let's get it done! This doesn't mean you suddenly become Superman, able to withstand any temptation—it just means avoiding it and delaying gratification becomes SUBSTANTIALLY easier.

# INTERVIEW WITH JASON GREY, VETERAN AND RETIRED FEDERAL LAW ENFORCEMENT OFFICER

Jason Grey is former military and a former federal agent. I chose to feature Jason in this chapter as I have benefited tremendously from Jason's wisdom and writing. Jason has also been through many difficult situations both professionally and personally, which has given him a very unique perspective on life that he can share with other people. And I asked Jason to talk specifically about discipline, as he lives and breathes it daily.

**Daniel Kelly:** Jason, tell us a bit about your background and training and how discipline became an integral part of your life.

**Jason Grey:** When high school came to an end, I had an idea of what I wanted to do in my life, but no straight arrow direction. College was the last thing I wanted to do, and I disliked any sort of academic environment. I figured the military would be a good move for a few reasons. First off, I knew that in some shape or form it would guarantee me a check for the rest of my life if I wanted it to. Second, I felt the pull of wanting to "do more" than just some normal job. That said, I had no one in my family in the military, and I didn't know a lot about it.

One day a friend of the family came by and said I should check out the reserves. I figured if I liked it, I could always go full time. Plus, after 9/11 it didn't seem to matter what unit you were in, there would always be work. So I joined and went through basic training. Anyone who has ever been in will say basic training or boot camp was a joke, but it wasn't a joke when you were in it. You learn to grow up real quick. Every button available on the human psyche is pushed—over and over again. It was not an easy transition, and in fact was a wake-up call.

In the military, no matter what your job is, you learn a few things. First, you learn death is very real and very quick. You come to terms with death (if you haven't already in your life), knowing it can happen at any time. The other thing you learn is discipline comes in many forms. And if you don't practice it, you could pay for it with your life. I was just a kid who landed in Afghanistan, but I quickly realized following directions (a form of discipline) was very important.

People often idealize a life of discipline, but they don't see the other side of it. The strong foundation I built while out on deployment didn't come without cost. No matter their job, everyone who comes back brings something home with them. When a human being is "on alert" for that amount of time, it changes them. That's not some cliché war quote, but turning it off is not always easy.

I did a few more stints on active duty and made it to sergeant. Then I called time on my career in the military and applied for jobs in the federal government. Tens of thousands apply for these jobs, and luckily, I got hired with a government agency working in counter-terrorism. The truth is when I got to training, I was surprised—and not in a good way. The training was over six months and was hardcore. The firearm part of the course was some of the toughest in the government and required extreme amounts of discipline.

In the beginning I didn't take it seriously enough and almost paid for it by not graduating. This forced me to better myself and led me on the path to self-improvement. At the time, my personal life was a complete wreck. My mind was not disciplined or focused enough on training. At one point they told me in no uncertain terms, if I didn't "un-fuck" myself, I was gone.

This was when the light bulb went off. I was letting my personal life ruin this amazing opportunity. This was a training school run off of extreme discipline and I wasn't practicing it. I remember going back to my room and laying on my bed for what seemed like hours. Then I finally concluded I would pass and I would un-fuck myself. The next day I took one of the final tests and passed it with a good score. What got me through was focusing once again on discipline and what it means, and I think everyone has to define what discipline means to them.

A person has to know discipline is not just blindly following orders or doing things "by the book" because someone says so. You have to have personal discipline, you have to know what it means to you. You have to have boundaries, but you have to know what they are. You have to be able to look at them objectively and use them to your advantage. Discipline is not a one-size-fits-all program. You must know how discipline works into your life and what it will do for you.

I took it too far sometimes, and it affected my personal life, ruining relationships and friendships. Although it wasn't discipline that was the problem, it was how I applied it. This is why I tell people to understand what discipline truly means because if you let it, it can run wild.

The same also applies to a lack of discipline—if you have none, it will run wild. For most of my jobs I had to be in good shape. That required discipline, especially when I was traveling all over the world. I had to know what discipline meant to me, and I had to know what my priorities were. This applies to all of us; **we have to know "why" we want to be disciplined**. We either take it seriously or we don't. It's that simple.

**Daniel Kelly:** You've been in dangerous, life-threatening situations. How did discipline help you succeed in those scenarios?

**Jason Grey:** There are tons of stories and close calls, situations most people will never be in, but none would make a Hollywood movie. Everything is subjective. There were many times I thought about things going wrong when I was working. The reality was, while terrorist attacks don't happen in the area I worked in everyday, they could happen. So I always needed to be aware and ready.

When you're in these situations, fear is definitely present. But you can't allow it to get the best of you. This is why you need mental discipline to be able to control your mind. I recall being on an outpost overseas and hearing what sounded like a gunshot near our gate. By the time I looked toward the sound and looked back up at my team, they were all standing there with M16s, SAWs, and whatever they could find. Everyone was ready. That may sound cool, but they needed to be ready; if someone came through that gate, it wouldn't have been so cool. I remember some of us "wishing" something would pop off, but I was always thinking in the back of my head that if it did we might lose someone. It's not like the movies.

Every job I've ever had was potentially dangerous—things could quickly go south. When I worked with the federal government, our training focused on doing things alone or in small teams. We were always told there would <u>never be backup</u>, and in our positions, there was no way there could be. You have to have a **massive amount of discipline** to be able to mentally handle that. While everyone is running out of the place, you're looking for the person trying to kill everyone.

In these roles you are told to rely on your training. In other words, you rely on discipline. You have a code and a set of rules; you rely on them and what you have trained for to get you through. When I was in dangerous situations, I was fortunate to always have confidence in what I knew. This is not to say I never messed up or didn't have some bumps along the way. But if you rely on your discipline and what you know, it will get you through. This is why people who are interviewed after shootings don't remember reacting. The adrenaline kicks in, and their response from the training and discipline is automatic.

**Daniel Kelly:** Why is discipline so important, and why is it so lacking in young men today?

**Jason Grey:** Having a foundation of discipline is key. Sadly, today most think discipline is optional, and people are raised without any discipline whatsoever. But you don't have to be in a life-threatening situation for discipline to work for you. It applies to everything. Without discipline you have no drive. To get a job you need discipline, to work out you need discipline, to go outside of your house you need discipline. In some shape or form, it plays a role in everything we do.

There are many reasons why discipline is lacking today. If you live in your mom's basement and text all day, what use is living a structured or disciplined lifestyle? When you've had everything given to you, you don't see the need for discipline. The path of least resistance is the best way for most, and that does not involve discipline.

But the flip side is, because discipline is so lacking, people are waking up to how necessary it is. Often you need extremes to see how bad something is. At this point it's almost a sport to write motivational quotes and pretend you're disciplined on the Internet yet do nothing of the sort in your own life. However, people with any real discipline see right through this. In our politically correct culture, where everything is based off emotion and has zero truth or reality, it's popular to be undisciplined. Merely suggesting someone isn't reaching their potential because they lack discipline is met with uproar.

Young men actually have to find the drive from within to become disciplined, or be around those who are. It's easier to not be disciplined and find comfort in being lazy. Society has built a safety net of unproductiveness by saying it's okay to be lazy.

**Daniel Kelly:** What concepts did you learn during your career that men can apply to their own lives?

**Jason Grey:** Things don't always go exactly as you want them to, although this doesn't mean things can't go good for you. You just need to realize life isn't going to cater to you.

Most of our issues, if not all of them, come from wanting something. We want something to go a certain way. So if it doesn't, then what? We lose our minds over the outcome. We waste our energy trying to think everything to death, or wondering why it didn't go the way we planned.

Have a plan and know what your goals are, but be okay if they don't turn out exactly how you want. I don't advocate you sit in a cave and meditate all day, or don't go after what you want. What I mean is, be okay with the outcome regardless of what that looks like. That's real power and control. In my career, there was not one situation that ever turned out the way I planned.

I recall being deployed and telling myself I could "think" my way out of any situation. Wrong. The better way to think about it is, *Yes, I do hold the answers to most of my questions.* Thinking about things won't make them better, but being okay with reality will. If there is a hurricane outside, your home will probably get damaged, so stop hoping it won't be. We have to live our lives with reality in mind, yet we don't.

The reason life doesn't go the "way we want" is because life is not designed around us. Once you realize that, life becomes a lot easier. This doesn't mean life is "against" us, but life is what it is. It took me

30 years to figure that out, but it's clear as day now. If I wake up tomorrow and say, "I hate birds," there will be 200 of them on my car when I walk outside. That's life. It's not being pessimistic—it's being realistic.

**Daniel Kelly:** One topic you are passionate about is hacks (i.e., the tendency of people to seek shortcuts instead of putting in the work). What do you think is the difference between a life of hacks and a life of discipline?

**Jason Grey:** Meditation, mindfulness, etc. only work for people aware enough to know what they are doing. If you take someone who has been in constant anxiety for 30 years and say, "Sit down and meditate," what do you think is going to happen? Hell, maybe they will become "enlightened" in one sitting. But the reality is they will probably go right back to their original patterns. Realistically, 30 years of neurological pathways are not going to be rebuilt in 20 minutes. Another example is when people take medications for depression but are still depressed. The change has to come from within. The mind is a powerful thing, but if you don't know how to control it, it will control you.

That's not to say nothing will ever work for you. There are plenty of tools to use when someone is actually in a position to use them. But most are not, and that's why they don't work. That's the issue. No one is doing anything for the journey—it's all what they can get out of it. They do it once and complain it didn't work for them. People go to seminars and scream they love themselves, jump up and down to music, or meditate and stay quiet for a week. But what happens when they get back on the airplane? All the old patterns return. As I reverted back to my training in my job, they revert back to their own "training." This is an important concept to understand if people want to permanently change their state.

As for books, most are way too long. They spend 400 pages trying to prove their stuff works, but all they do is give you little mental tricks to induce a happy state for five minutes. Most authors sell books to drone on about something that could be explained in 50 pages. However, knowing how to apply things to your situation is what works. You have to look at your problems like an onion and work through the layers. When you go through the layers, you eventually get to the source. Now it's all in front of you. **That's the "hack" right there.**

# CHAPTER 15

# BALANCE AND SPIRITUALITY

Most Westerners view spirituality as some woo woo concept dreamt up by crackpots, religious zealots, and New Age gurus. And I get it. The reason many are alienated by spirituality is that it appears so abstract. Although, you don't have to be a Tibetan monk meditating in a cave every day to be spiritual. Since time immemorial, spirituality has been an integral part of human existence. We have always had a desire to find greater meaning and purpose. To truly reach your full potential as a man, you must optimize your mind, body, *and* spirit. And to unite these three elements is the highest calling of every man.

What does hormone optimization have to do with spirituality? We are energetic beings—indeed, the yogic traditions affirm we have seven energetic centers in our bodies known as "chakras." So when you enhance your health through hormone optimization, these energetic centers become aligned. Now, I don't have a study to back this up, but I've lost count of the number of people whose lives found deeper meaning once they got into peak condition and optimized their hormones. In my own case, my perspective on life radically changed once I underwent testosterone replacement therapy.

But what if you don't care about spirituality? That's cool. I encourage you to read through this chapter nevertheless to see if anything resonates with you. In this chapter, you will find some ideas and practices you can incorporate into your life to help you develop a deeper sense of self. Because, ultimately, what are you doing all this for? We earn money, improve our health, seek relationships, etc., mostly because we want to feel better about ourselves. And one surefire way to feel better about yourself is to practice some of the things we discuss here.

## YOUR EGO AND PRACTICING NON-JUDGMENT

Nowadays, there's a lot of talk about "ego." But what really is the ego? *The Collins Dictionary* provides an ample definition, "Someone's ego is their sense of their own worth. For example, if someone has a large ego, they think they are very important and valuable."[267] Your ego is the little voice in your head that's always seeking conflict. **Its default state is us versus them**. Your ego is what wants to start fights because it feels insulted. Your ego is the urge to interrupt others and get your point across because it needs to be "right." Your ego is what gets pissed when someone cuts you off in traffic.

But the real you—not your ego—is a spiritual being that has far more in common with others than it does differences. However, your ego doesn't want you to know this. It wants to protect its survival, so it perpetuates a state of conflict and division. Now you may rightly ask—what is the point of the ego, if all it does is cause problems?

The answer is, the ego is not entirely pointless. It's primarily responsible for keeping us alive and developing our personality. Once you start to become aware of the ego in your daily life, you realize how much of your life is driven by it. And when you become conscious of it, you no longer identify with it and remain a slave to it. Then you are well on the way to self-mastery.

***One can have no smaller or greater mastery than mastery of oneself. —Leonardo da Vinci***

---

267   *Collins Dictionary, s.v.,* "Ego," accessed January 9, 2019, https://www.collinsdictionary.com/us/dictionary/english/ego.

A practice I've found useful for keeping the ego in a healthy place is that of non-judgment. Everything we do on a daily basis involves some form of judgment or labeling. For example, imagine you're walking down the street and you see an attractive girl in a dress and think, "She's cute!" Or you see an overweight guy in a restaurant shoveling food into his mouth and you say to yourself, "Man, that guy is fat!" Or perhaps you're at the gym and you see a guy doing an exercise with horrendous form and think, "What an idiot!" These judgments and labels do nothing for us, and they only serve to further entrench us in the world of ego.

Now, imagine the scenarios above once more, but this time try not to pass judgment. For instance, you see the girl in the street and you take in her beauty all the same. But now you simply appreciate it, without the need to label it or have a conversation in your mind. You see the same guy at the restaurant—and maybe he is eating a lot. But why should it bother you—is it because it goes against social norms of acceptable behavior? Or perhaps it irritates your ego, and not *you*? Try sitting and observing instead of judging.

Thoughts will still come into your head and you'll still think the same things. They don't just disappear—but the difference between judgment and non-judgment is whether you acknowledge the thoughts or not. This practice is a radical concept for most people, simply because we're so used to labeling everything. Don't worry if it's hard at first—you are changing a lifelong habit, after all. But when you begin to put this into practice, you will have more compassion and empathy for people, where before you felt scorn or disdain for people because your ego was always judging them. In my own case, there are times when I forget to do this and resort back to judging and labeling everything. However, when I make a conscious effort to focus on this practice, I have greater peace of mind because I no longer pay attention to the endless chatter of the voice in my head.

## MAKE DEATH YOUR CONSTANT COMPANION

If you examine your fears and worries under a microscope, you will see at the heart of most is the fear of death. Common fears such as finances, job security, growing old, or your health are what I call "surface worries." These things are cause for concern, but they are not the real reason you're worried. We need to go a few levels deeper.

For example, you worry about your finances or job security because if you have no money, you won't be able to pay the bills. If you don't pay your bills, you may go into debt and struggle to make payments, and eventually you'll be out on the street. If you're on the street, you'll struggle to feed yourself and your family, and you'll starve to death. As you can see from this exercise, it wasn't finances or job security that was the real issue—it was the fear of death. Most people don't realize this because they've never taken the time to examine their thoughts for what they really are.

I used to constantly worry about my health. It even has its own term: *health anxiety*. I would monitor every ache and pain in my body and would convince myself I was developing a disease. From a brain tumor, to heart disease, to testicular cancer—I was convinced I had them all. It all seems quite ridiculous now, but at the time, I truly believed I had to anticipate any disease, so I had the best chance of fighting it. Yet all along, it wasn't the fear of disease that was the problem. The reason I feared the disease was because I feared death.

**The day you accept your own death is the day you become free.** Knowing you can depart this world at any moment and being okay with it is true freedom. It's counterintuitive, but it actually gives you a greater sense of inner peace. Most people pretend as if death is never going to happen. People avoid thinking about it because it scares them so much. Ironically, this is why they never pursue their dreams—because they have no sense of urgency over their own death. So they aren't compelled to take action. The shortness of life and imminence of death can energize you instead of paralyzing you. This is illustrated by a passage in the brilliant book, *King, Warrior, Magician, Lover*, which I highly recommend. The authors describe how warriors throughout history used the awareness of death to empower them to live exceptional lives:

> The Warrior traditions all affirm that, in addition to training, what enables a Warrior to reach clarity of thought is living with the awareness of his own imminent death. The Warrior knows the shortness of life and how fragile it is. A man under the guidance of the Warrior knows how few his days are.
>
> Rather than depressing him, this leads to an outpouring of life force and to an intense experience of life that is unknown to others. Every act counts. Each deed is done as if it were the last. The samurai swordsmen were taught to live their lives as if they were already dead. Castaneda's Don Juan taught that there is "no time" for anything but meaningful acts if we are to live with death as "our eternal companion."[268]

*Like the generations of leaves, the lives of mortal men. Now the wind scatters the old leaves across the earth, now the living timber bursts with the new buds and spring comes round again. And so with men: as one generation comes to life, another dies away. —Homer, The Iliad*

When you accept your own death, there will be few things you cannot confront. Because if you accept death, what else is there to be afraid of? In my case, once I acknowledged I was more than my mind and body (i.e., a spiritual being), it was much easier to accept

---

268 Robert Moore and Doug Gillette. *King, Warrior, Magician, Lover: Rediscovering the Archetypes of the Mature Masculine* (HarperOne, 2013).

death because I recognized my life on Earth was merely one part of my existence. It was no coincidence that I was able to embrace this idea fully once I optimized my hormones and my physical health. That's why I truly believe you cannot become the best version of yourself unless you take care of your body. The clarity of thought and purpose that optimal testosterone levels provided allowed me to let go and come to terms with it. What might you be able to accomplish when you accept your own death?

## MEDITATION AND MINDFULNESS

The earliest references to meditation come from ancient India around 1500 BCE. It's been around for a long time, but only in recent decades has it started to gain popularity in the Western world. For most, the idea of meditation invokes images of sitting on a mat with your eyes closed. However, in reality there are many forms of meditation, and you don't have to sit in silence to be in a meditative state.

One form of meditation that I like is mindfulness. Essentially, mindfulness is the practice of being aware in the present moment. So instead of running on autopilot, becoming lost in your thoughts—as most of us do—you devote your entire concentration to your present activity. That means almost any activity can become meditative.

For example, lifting weights is meditation; you feel the muscle contractions with each repetition and become one with your body. Walking in the mountains can be meditation; breathing in the fresh air and experiencing the stillness and serenity of nature. The ultimate goal here is to quiet the mind. Indeed, you can achieve this through traditional meditation. However, many people don't have the time or inclination to do this. You can achieve similar results by practicing mindfulness and becoming aware in the present moment.

When you quiet the mind, **you realize you are not your mind.** When you experience stillness, free of thoughts, you access a level of consciousness and knowing beyond your conscious mind. This helps you realize you are more than just your body. And once you've tasted it, you will never go back to your old way of thinking.

I aim to practice traditional meditation for 10–15 minutes daily. But above all, my goal is to be mindful in every activity I do. My morning routine typically consists of journaling, breathing, and contemplation; these are all meditative for me. Do what works for you. Meditate while sitting on a mat, apply mindfulness to your daily life—or do both.

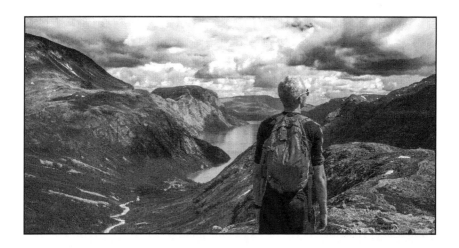

## NO FAP

"No Fap" is a concept that has become increasingly popular with Millennials in recent times. No Fap is the practice of abstaining from pornography, masturbation, and even sex for a period of time. Although abstaining from sex altogether is a bit extreme—like a religion that advocates the repression of sexual desires. Nonetheless, abstaining from masturbation, and *especially* porn, can be very beneficial for you.

But why talk about No Fap in a book on hormone optimization? Because as a man, your sexual energy is one of the most powerful forces in the universe. Think about it; your sperm is literally what creates life. Consider how compelling your desire is when you see an attractive woman—you feel the energy surge through your body. And when our sexual desire is harnessed in a positive way, it moves mountains. This is what Napoleon Hill termed "sexual transmutation."

But when sexual desire is channeled for the wrong reasons, it can be toxic and destructive. We've all jacked off to porn and felt the dopamine rush from it, only to feel empty and often disgusted immediately after. The stark reality is quite disturbing: in a similar manner to substance abuse, porn addiction can actually rewire parts of your brain, resulting in more poor judgment and impulsive and aggressive behavior.[269]

I can already hear your disapproval, "But I need to jack off, otherwise I'll go crazy!" True, the desire to have sex is strong for most men, so they think they need a release. The reality is, most men have never learned how to harness the power of their sexual energy, and they let it control them. The only reason men think they constantly need a sexual release is because porn is so freely available. In our culture, sex is on every corner. Do you think your grandfather spent his days jerking off? Of course not; he had to go out and provide for his family. This is how our civilization was built. Industry was created on the backs of men who harnessed their sexual desire in a positive way. If you jack off to porn all day, you can't possibly harness your sexual energy.

---

269   Donald L. Hilton, Jr and Clark Watts, "Pornography addiction: A neuroscience perspective," *Surg Neurol Int*, 2011, 2: 19, published online 2011 Feb 21, doi: 10.4103/2152-7806.76977.

What has jerking off to porn ever done for you? All because monkey brain wants its dopamine fix, but how do you know you can't resist it? And more besides, what will you feel like, and what might you be capable of, when you do resist it? If you don't know, try it and see what happens. Try taking a week off porn and see how you feel. This will force you to go out and talk to REAL women!

Masturbation is just a habit like anything else, and that means it can be broken. Ditch the cues that make you jack off (e.g., boredom or being alone). Instead, go out and take action. Go to the gym, play a sport, or read a book. Oftentimes in life, it's not what you can do more of, it's what you can do less of. I guarantee you will feel better for it—you'll have more energy, more concentration, and better self-esteem.

We live in an intellect-dominant culture that basically denies the existence of spirituality. However, we are multifaceted beings, so it stands to reason that there are multiple aspects to our health. Spirituality is a fundamental aspect of your health that you cannot afford to neglect. Proper exercise and nutrition alone cannot fill the hole in a life devoid of spirituality. Begin with the ideas described in this chapter. If the topic resonates with you, explore more books on the subject. Now join me to read the case studies of young men who underwent TRT.

# CHAPTER 16

# CASE STUDIES: YOUNG MEN ON TESTOSTERONE

The choice to undergo testosterone therapy is a big decision at any age. It means you're going to be reliant on a medication, and possibly inject yourself, for the rest of your life. Such decisions can't be made at the drop of a hat. This decision is also made more difficult in a day and age where there is so much misinformation about testosterone. Is it safe? Is it as good as they say it is? Will I become infertile? It's natural to have questions and even trepidation about this decision.

We've talked a lot about the science behind hormone optimization and why increasing your testosterone levels is so beneficial. Academic studies and research are one thing, but there is no substitution for firsthand accounts of men who've actually undergone testosterone replacement therapy themselves at such a young age. When you read someone's personal story, you see that they often have the same doubts and insecurities you do. You can relate to them, and that reassures you to know you're not the only one going through this plight.

Whenever I need more information to make a decision, I always take into consideration the firsthand experiences of others. In this chapter we'll hear the stories of men, including myself, who underwent testosterone optimization at a young age.

## THE RELIGION OF SCIENCE: SHOW ME THE STUDY

One thing that has become readily apparent in our society is how science has become the new religion of the 21st century. For reasons beyond the scope of this book, religion in the West has ceased to play a central role in our lives. As the saying goes, nature abhors a vacuum, and this vacuum has now been filled by science.

Science plays a prominent role in our daily lives. Science has empowered us with knowledge and objective truths about reality. According to science skeptic Michael Shermer, science is "a set of methods designed to describe and interpret observed or inferred phenomena, past or present, aimed at building a testable body of knowledge open to rejection or confirmation."[270] As a result, we no longer blindly follow religious dogma and superstition. However, today we appear to have veered toward the other end of the spectrum, where science has become a religion unto itself. It believes itself to be *the* truth. And if science doesn't validate it, it doesn't exist.

This "show me the study" mindset extends to testosterone replacement therapy. The same individuals refute anecdotal stories on the benefits of testosterone. But the fact that millions of men all around the world are successfully using testosterone is proof positive that it works, yet these people still cling to the toxic mindset that a study is required for anything to be credible. Sadly, they fail to see that their revered "scientific" studies can be skewed and manipulated to obtain desired outcomes. And oftentimes they are funded by parties with a conflict of interest who are invested in the outcome of the study.

Clinical research is an important part of making informed decisions on your health. Indeed, this book itself relies heavily on science. I'm not saying you should accept everything put in front of you, but

---

270  Michael Shermer, *Why Darwin Matters: The Case Against Intelligent Design* (Macmillan, 2007).

you should also understand studies have flaws. It's your job to think critically and discern things for YOURSELF.

*The declining health and wellness of our society is due, in large part, to adherence to the inherently flawed principles shrouded within the "scientific method." Always question the assumptions within. —Dr. Merrill Matschke*

## JOSHUA BAKHUN

I remember it like it was yesterday—it was another Saturday night sitting home. Here I was, 29 years old, and once again, I had zero motivation to socialize. The thing is, I always had a good social circle and girlfriends over the years, but now I had turned into a recluse. And in truth, I didn't really want to be around *anyone*.

On paper things looked good: I had a good six-figure income, I was in the prime of life, and I was in decent shape. Yet, I had no desire to live the life of a healthy adult! How could I possibly be at the lowest point of my life when I had no major problems?

One day, in a haze of depression I found myself scrolling through Facebook and came across one of my acquaintances, Jay Campbell. Not only did he have a physique I very much envied, but he was killing it in his career and social life as well. So in my desperation, I sent him a message. I needed change, and this was my last throw of the dice.

He recommended I get blood work done, and he put me in touch with a doctor to assess the results. Once I got the results back, I sat down with the doctor, who told me I had low testosterone. What? How could I have low testosterone? I always worked out and tried to eat correctly. I'm only 29! Could this even be possible?

However, I realized I was not alone in my ordeal and that other young men were suffering from similar issues. I was hesitant to start testosterone therapy, though, because I knew it was a lifelong commitment. Injecting myself for the rest of my life wasn't something I could mentally grasp. So I decided I would try it for two months and see how I felt. If I didn't feel different then I would quit and look for another solution. Needless to say, after four weeks into testosterone therapy, I knew I would never look back.

The turnaround was incredible. Not only had I put on a decent amount of muscle and lost body fat, but I was socializing again and dating new girls weekly! And I don't believe it was a coincidence I received a major job promotion as a result of my massive drive and effort. My life literally changed before my eyes, and other people started to notice too. My mom called me one day and asked me what I had been doing differently. She said I seemed happy for the first time in a while, and whatever it was, I should "keep it up!"

## JASON GREY

Years of government work had taken its toll on my mind and body, and I knew something had to change. After reading Jay Campbell's TRT Manual, I decided to get my blood work checked. The results of the blood work showed someone overworked and overstressed. I had the testosterone of an 80-year-old, and overall, I felt like crap.

I was put on a TRT regimen by the doctor at the clinic, and within a couple of weeks I felt like a new person. After three months, it wasn't even comparable to how I felt before. Sleep, which had always been a huge issue of mine, was now better along with stress. Hormone replacement allows the body to perform in a peak state, which makes anything to do with mood or the mind better.

The only way to describe post-TRT is a new overall context of what a man should feel like. It's very easy to "suck it up" for years when it comes to suboptimal hormones, but that will only go so far. Plus, the environment we live in is becoming more toxic and degenerate by the day; we have to fight against that. TRT puts a man where he is *supposed to be* hormonally. Sadly, most men don't know what the real normal feels like and go years without help.

As I said, the way I feel now is not comparable to before TRT. My energy is always on point along with my libido. Men on TRT feel more stable and balanced in their daily lives. This just puts you in the right kind of frame and mindset to accomplish what needs to be done anytime, anyplace. **Anyone serious about optimal performance, mentally and physically, should have their blood work done by a properly trained hormone expert.** And it might come as a surprise to see what comes back.

# INTERVIEW WITH MICHAEL KOCSIS

Michael is the founder of Balance My Hormones (balancemyhormones. co.uk) and has over 22 years of personal experience as a patient of testosterone replacement therapy. He holds a master's degree in business with a special focus on health care administration. He worked in pharmaceuticals, medical, surgical, and healthcare IT sales prior to starting his business. After an abrupt end to employment and a frustration with the lack of viable treatment options in the UK, Michael decided to pursue a dream of starting a successful hormone optimization service in the UK.

**Daniel Kelly:** Michael, you began testosterone therapy in your early 20s, at a time when testosterone treatment was still in its infancy. Tell us about your story of undergoing TRT and the challenges you faced.

**Michael Kocsis:** When I was 22, I began to think something wasn't quite right. I had all the typical symptoms associated with low T. I went to my family practice doctor and asked if he could order me a test. Yet, I will never forget the conversation, or should I say lecture, I was given. He told me not to "go down that path" and that testosterone would shorten my life and cause heart and prostate issues. He refused to even offer a blood test. Ultimately, I found a partially understanding private doctor who was reluctantly willing to prescribe me testosterone.

In those days, it was common practice to see the doctor every two weeks for an injection of testosterone enanthate with a small dose of testosterone propionate and vitamin B12. Although I was a bit cheeky and would arrive a week early so my injection would be every seven days, as opposed to the two-week regimen that left me feeling suboptimal.

After 120 days, he said it was time to come off testosterone. His theory was that my natural testosterone would increase through exogenous injections, and then my body would remember this new level after he slowly weaned me off. Sadly, this doctor didn't understand basic endocrinology, and this obviously didn't work. His theory left me with lower testosterone levels than when I started— even after a year without TRT.

After seeing numerous endocrinologists and being treated as if I were addicted to testosterone, I finally met a doctor in California who was far ahead of his time, and he put me on a proper treatment protocol. Young men have it easier today, especially in North America, as there are more and more TRT centers offering options for them that I didn't have at the time.

**Daniel Kelly:** You've used testosterone patches, gels, and injections over the years. What was your experience with them, and what in your opinion is the best form of treatment as a patient?

**Michael Kocsis:** When I finally found an endocrinologist willing to treat me after the first GP stopped treatment, he decided the best option was testosterone patches. He told me I had to wear two at a time. The patches did help, as the testosterone was slowly absorbed into my body. Although, it was quite awkward to wear them, and I felt very self-conscious.

I never used gels, as they were inferior to what I was offered by the Californian doctor. He had a patent on a bespoke cream called Testocreme®. It was a special formulation of high-concentration cream in a highly absorbable base in a hybrid cream/gel form. It worked very well, and after using it for the first time, I noticed a surge of energy and morning erections.

Sometime in the early 2000s, I began seeing a new doctor who recommended injectable testosterone cypionate. I remained on that formulation until around 2011, when I made the switch to Sustanon at 125 mg every five days. Sustanon works perfectly for me, and my trough levels (i.e., a blood test five days after injection) are in the top end of the normal range—around 923 ng/dL (32 nmol/L), which is ideal. I am also prescribed hCG at 500 IU, which I take 2–3 times per week, in addition to 0.5 mg of anastrozole per week. It took some experimentation with my doctor, but I find these doses and this combination of medications allows me to feel my best.

**Daniel Kelly:** In your experience, what are the most common concerns young men have about TRT, and are their fears justified?

**Michael Kocsis:** Many young men are afraid of the prospect that they will be dependent on testosterone for life. I find it ironic that this isn't a problem if you're diabetic and need insulin. A growing trend with testosterone is that it's something you do for a short time and stop. Although, this is probably the worst thing you can do.

The underlying cause of this anxiety may be the fear of not being able to maintain a supply of testosterone throughout one's life. The doctor in California told me I would always have testosterone. I don't think he meant he would always be my doctor, but rather if you see testosterone as the foundation to everything, you will find a way to make sure your supply doesn't run out.

What's the alternative—remain suboptimal for the rest of your life? Some young men I speak to are fearful of losing their hair. But this only happens if you are genetically prone to it. The other issue some men have is a lack of understanding, or pressure from partners not to start TRT. I've had some men tell me they couldn't go through with treatment because their partner said it was either them or the testosterone.

There is a lack of understanding among the general population about testosterone. Some view testosterone as cosmetic, rather than to promote health and well-being, so many partners are suspicious about it for this reason. Funnily enough, some partners even fear they may not be able to keep up with their man's reinvigorated libido! Therefore, people who claim they are looking out for their partner's welfare are just trying to cover their own inadequacies. Another fear that comes up is shrinking testes, and this is easily remedied if the doctor prescribes hCG.

**Daniel Kelly:** Using exogenous testosterone shuts down your body's own production of testosterone, which diminishes fertility, as endogenous testosterone is key to sperm production. You were on testosterone for many years before taking hCG. How has this affected your fertility?

**Michael Kocsis:** When I first started, I only was prescribed exogenous testosterone. I was also prescribed anastrozole as my estrogen (E2) had elevated, which raised my prolactin levels. The doctor recommended adding an AI to lower estrogen, and by doing so, he said prolactin would come down—and it did. Being in the sweet spot with E2 and testosterone may have helped keep the size of my testes stable. One endocrinologist warned me my testicles would shrink to the size of raisins if I stayed on TRT. That never happened to me.

I can't tell you for sure what my fertility was after almost 20 years on TRT and brief experimentations with hCG. After 18 months of TRT with hCG and low dose anastrozole, my sperm count is over 156 million with 72% motility, and this is well above what is needed for fertility (20 million). So despite 20 years of testosterone and a mild varicocele, the addition of hCG has allowed me to maintain my fertility.

**Daniel Kelly:** After being a patient of testosterone in both the US and UK, how does the approach toward treatment differ in these countries?

**Michael Kocsis:** When I began TRT, it was like the Dark Ages in the US. Transdermal patches were a new concept. The pitch was that it was easy to use, which meant you could avoid injections. This opened up the treatment to men who could easily apply a topical patch from the comfort of their homes without having to see a doctor for an injection. It was difficult to find a doctor in the Midwest in the late 1990s with enough of an understanding, hence why I sought treatment in California, where it was more advanced.

The US has a private insurance-base model, which can dictate to the doctor the type of treatment offered by refusing to pay for certain treatments. If you have good insurance coverage from your employer, your doctor in that network may be more amenable to prescribing treatment. But it really depends what the insurance covers.

I had a friend in Atlanta who was refused an aromatase inhibitor, despite his estradiol (E2) being off the charts and found it very frustrating. I, on the other hand, had a preferred provider organization (PPO), and my prescribing doctor had no issue with recommending an AI. So it can be a bit of a lottery. I was fortunate to come across more open-minded doctors in the US who eventually helped fine-tune my treatment.

The UK today, especially with the NHS (National Healthcare Service), seems to be in a similar state as the US in the late 1990s, with the exception of a few thought leaders in the UK, including the doctors I work with. In the UK, I found the NHS to be a national treasure, but disappointing when it comes to TRT. I felt like I had gone back in time with their available treatment options.

They wanted me to go in for injections of Nebido (Aveed), or inject Sustanon every three weeks! In addition, hCG was not on offer, nor was an AI. Frankly, I was horrified and annoyed, as everything was in balance before I went to see them, and their outdated practices jeopardized it. The NHS restrictive guidelines and "computer says no" mentality seems to be based more around cost-cutting and austerity than a bespoke approach, as with the US. When I looked at the private side, I couldn't be sure who would be open-minded and knowledgeable enough in the field. Thankfully, I eventually managed to find a compassionate, open-minded doctor to prescribe me medication.

# CHAPTER 17

# THE FINAL WORD—HOW TO RECLAIM YOUR MASCULINITY

If you've got this far, it means you've taken the time to read and absorb everything in this book. However, in this day and age our problem is not that we lack information. In fact, with the Internet, we have more than we could ever dream of. Our problem is we are spoiled for choice—information overload. As a result, we end up with analysis paralysis. Do yourself a favor and take action on the lessons you've learned in this book. You don't have to do it all at once, but just do something.

I already know that if you're reading this book then you're into self-development, and that's fantastic because I share your passion. However, I've been around the self-development genre long enough to know it's easy to fool yourself that you're taking action. But in reality, you're not. Reading books and listening to podcasts and audiobooks is great, although consuming a boatload of content is just another form of procrastination in disguise. To reclaim your masculinity, you must become a man of action.

When I find myself consuming too much information and not taking enough action, I recall the story of when Henry Ford brought a lawsuit against a Chicago newspaper for defamation. After a long line of questioning and offensive statements, Ford became exasperated and exclaimed:

> If I should really WANT to answer the foolish question you have just asked, or any of the other questions you have been asking me, let me remind you that I have a row of electric

push-buttons on my desk. And by pushing the right button, I can summon to my aid men who can answer ANY question I desire concerning the business to which I am devoting most of my efforts. Now, will you kindly tell me, WHY I should clutter up my mind with general knowledge, for the purpose of being able to answer questions, when I have men around me who can supply any knowledge I require?[271]

Remember this when you find yourself needlessly cluttering your own mind.

## TESTOSTERONE AND PURPOSE

When you optimize your hormones, an amazing thing happens. As a snake sheds its skin, you shed the shackles of anxiety, indecisiveness, and fear. It's as though you can see clearly for the first time. Suddenly, your life takes on a whole new meaning. You become razor focused on your goals. You summon courage to go after what you've always wanted. No motivational hacks required. This is how nature intended you to be as a man: be bold, powerful, and strong.

Optimal testosterone has the power to transform you into a man of action. Men constructed civilizations, traveled to the moon, and built everything you see around you. This is your birthright as a man, but it's up to you to claim it. Every man in history who accomplished anything great went and claimed it for himself. You cannot just sit at home and hope that fame, fortune, and a hot girl will land on your lap. You must go out and get them. This is the testosterone mindset. The universe does not reward men for wishful thinking and daydreaming. However, the universe does conspire to help men who take action and live life with purpose.

271 "Henry Ford was the smartest ignorant man in history," 500 Dollar Millionaire, June 26, 2013, https://500dollarmillionaire.wordpress.com/2013/06/26/henry-ford-was-the-smartest-ignorant-man-in-history/.

Yet today many young men are confused about their purpose in life. But understand, your purpose will not come by trawling Google or watching motivational videos on YouTube. Just like money and women won't suddenly land in your lap, nor will your purpose. Stop worrying about finding your purpose all the time, and stop looking to things outside of you to light the fire within you. The best chance of discovering your purpose is by living a full and varied life. And you do this by focusing on your health, and in particular your hormonal balance. The ultimate irony is, when you stop trying to find your purpose, it finds you.

## THE PRICE OF HEALTH

I hope by now you realize how important hormonal balance and overall health is to you as a man. Sadly, many men still fail to prioritize their health. They make up excuses:

"I don't have time."
"TRT is too expensive."
<Insert other excuses here>

In life there's always a price to pay; whether it's time-related, monetary, or emotional. Truth be told, it doesn't cost much to look after your health. In fact, research suggests low testosterone can cost you a lot of money because of all the mental health problems and medical bills associated with it.[272]

If you think a few hundred dollars a month is too much to pay for your health, you have got your priorities SERIOUSLY wrong. You need to see your health as an investment because the ROI it has is exponential. Think about it—how much do you spend each

---

272   Huanguang Jia, Charles T Sullivan, Sean C McCoy, Joshua F Yarrow, Matthew Morrow, and Stephen E Borst, "Review of health risks of low testosterone and testosterone administration," *World J Clin Cases*, 2015 Apr 16, 3(4): 338–344, published online 2015 Apr 16, doi: 10.12998/wjcc.v3.i4.338.

month on alcohol, restaurants, entertainment, and other bullshit? Yet nutritious food, going to the gym, or even testosterone is too expensive?

All it means is that your health is not a priority. If your health were in jeopardy, you'd find a way and MAKE IT HAPPEN. In reality, if you're not looking after your health every day, then it is in jeopardy. You're just not in intensive care or lying six feet under yet, so you don't recognize the fact.

If a man has cancer, he would do ANYTHING to try and rid himself of it. Yet, many men still haven't grasped the fact that low testosterone is *not* optional. **It's not a benign condition—it's just as deadly and serious as cancer or heart disease.** Perhaps it's because of the stigma around testosterone or just not knowing how to solve the issue. But now you have my book in your hands, you have no excuse.

# INTERVIEW WITH ANDREW TATE

Andrew Tate is an American-British kickboxer from Chicago, Illinois, who competes in the cruiserweight and heavyweight divisions. He is three times ISKA Kickboxing world champion and Enfusion Live champion, and is the son of the late chess master Emory Tate. He is well known for his outspoken views, particularly on the topics of masculinity and relationships. His raw honesty and authenticity is refreshing in a world where people don't speak their mind.

**Daniel Kelly:** Andrew, you've been crowned world kickboxing champion three times, can you talk a little bit about the mindset required to become a world champion?

**Andrew Tate:** Actually, it almost happened by accident. I was a professional chess player when I was a kid, and my dad was a professional chess player. So I was being trained to be a world-level chess player. I won the Indiana State Chess Championships at age five in the under 10s and was on my way to becoming a grandmaster. Then my mom and dad broke up and we moved to England. There was no chess scene there, so I decided I wanted to do something else. And to me, fighting and chess were quite similar. People think they're not, but they're both 1-on-1, it's still war, there's no team and there's no luck involved, so to me the parallels were evident.

Fighting is a perfection-sport. You know you could be a football player and drop the ball sometimes, but still be a good player. You can't be a good fighter and fuck up. You mess up and that's the end of it. Not just the end of the fight, but the end of your career and the end of your life. It's not a joke, so you have to dedicate yourself to understand you're never going to be good enough. You're never going to master or completely understand it, but you just keep going regardless.

My coach was a badass, an ex-special forces type—not to be fucked with. When I would walk into the gym with an injury and say, "I can't do that today," or "I'm tired," he'd say, "Do you think your opponent is going to go easier on you in a few weeks because today you're tired? Do you think if you say, "That hurts," or "I can't train," that your opponent is going to punch you any less in the face? He doesn't give a fuck about you. He's out to kill you. This is war, you've got to train. You've got to fight to survive." That was the mindset instilled into me from day one.

To be honest, I never said to myself I *would* be world champion, I just kept training and I'd fight anyone. I won my first world title on three days' notice. Someone else got injured, and they called me up. I was out of shape, and I had to lose 9 kg. I was like, "Fuck it!" I got home, I didn't eat, I spent time in the sauna, and I lost the weight. Then I got in there and I won. That's just how it all worked out. The mindset is very much just about realism. Your opponent is going to do their best to incapacitate me, and the only person that can save me is myself. That's what I loved about chess. That's what I love about fighting—it's individualism.

The only person who wakes up in the morning and says, "I'm going to make sure Andrew's life is amazing," is Andrew. There's no other motherfucker on this planet waking up saying, "I want to put money in Andrew's bank today." No one's doing that for me! The only person that can do that is me, so when people remove the individualism from their mind and they start blaming other people, understand: no one's going to improve your life but you. That's what fighting taught me—no one's going to win it for you.

**Daniel Kelly:** What are the parallels between the chess and kickboxing?

**Andrew Tate:** Chess is one of the only games you play with no luck, whereas with gambling or poker, for example, there is an element of luck involved. In chess, it's you against them, and it's fair. Perhaps black has a slight disadvantage because they go second, but in general it's a fair game—and if you lose, it's because you fucked up. It's really that simple; you cannot lose a game of chess without making a mistake.

Chess is very much like life—there's no move you can make without counterbalance. Even if it's the most perfect move in the world, there are always disadvantages. Even if they're miniscule, they exist; and life's the same. It doesn't matter what you decide to do, even if you decide to live the perfect life—I'm going to get up at this time, I'm going to train, etc.—there's a whole bunch of counterbalance you're missing out on. You're missing out on partying, the girls, or whatever. So chess is very balanced like that. Now kickboxing is the same, fighting is the same; it's you against them, and there's no luck. People say, "Lucky punch!" But there's no such thing as a lucky punch!

If you're fighting at world level, that guy has trained to punch people in the face for years and then he punches you in the face and knocks you out. Is that luck? That's not luck. There's no such thing as a lucky punch. It's absolute individualism, its 1-on-1, and it's war, because that's all sports are. They are watered down versions of war—that's why men play sports. Men used to go to war. It never used to be sports. They used to go around, find people who didn't look exactly the same as them, and fight them. That's how humans were. Now we have football and all kind of sports—it's all just different versions of war.

**Daniel Kelly:** In the past, you've said how men have an innate desire to conquer that they must embrace to feel truly happy. How can men fulfill this need for conquest in everyday life, and what happens if they deny it?

**Andrew Tate:** If you deny your instinct to conquer, you will become depressed and miserable. There's a lot of talk about the human condition and people try to dig into the whys. I'm not so much of a why-guy—I'm more of "this is how I am." This is how we evolved because the men who didn't think this way got their asses kicked and got killed. Men are designed to conquer. But when I say that, people think I'm talking about running around raping, committing crime, etc. I'm not talking about that. I'm talking about having something in your life that requires 100% focused effort for achievement.

It's the reason men are obsessed with their business, their job, or obsessed like the Wall Street guys who are on the phone for 15 hours a day. It's because they're looking to conquer the world. They don't give a shit about Wall Street—they don't even give a shit about whatever they sell. It's financial conquest. It's conquest just like any other.

People completely misunderstood me and started saying, "You're advocating rape. These ain't caveman days!" But once again, I'm not saying that. I'm saying you need to conquer the Earth in whichever sphere you find most relevant. Financial is one example, but it could be lots of things—even if you just conquer yourself. Conquer your body. Discipline yourself. Train when you don't want to train. Run when you don't want to run. There are a million different ways you can conquer your life, but when people refuse to do that, they end up just sorry sacks sitting on Twitter saying how you're wrong.

I know some very rich guys who lead entertaining lives, but there's no conquest in it, and they're not happy. I know some guys who have unlimited finance and they're bored and miserable. Then I know guys who earn a fraction of that, but they're hustling to get it, and they enjoy it. And we all know the old adage, "You don't appreciate it unless you earn it." Run your own little empire—we can't all be

Julius Caesar—but have your own shit going on. Your own house, your own car, your own woman, your own team. Get your own little empire together and you're going to be a happy individual. And that's why I say depression isn't real. Depression isn't real because your situation is shit. You haven't got disease; your situation's shit. Change your situation.

**Daniel Kelly:** In a recent interview, you said depression isn't real, and you got a lot of backlash from it. Can you elaborate on what you meant?

**Andrew Tate:** The way depression is currently understood is that it's this big evil monster that can come out of nowhere. And no matter how good your life is, it can strike you down. Now you're depressed and miserable, and your life is over! That's garbage. Depression is a situation. You don't need to look further than prison for proof. If depression wasn't situational, people wouldn't be afraid of going to prison. A prison will get you depressed because it's shit, and your situation is shit. But when you leave jail, all of a sudden, you're no longer depressed. That shows that depression is not some disease.

If you're unhappy with your situation, then change it. Although, you can only lead a horse to water. If you're going to refuse to improve your situation and improve your life, then you're going to continue to stay depressed. There are young men out there who say, "I'm depressed" because they're fat, have no girlfriend, or have no money. And they think the answer is mind-altering drugs, as opposed to getting a girlfriend and getting some money! It's crazy. Yet when I said that, I was ostracized and was in national papers in England, and everyone ripped me to pieces.

Writer Johann Hari has since spoken on depression and said the exact same thing I said. And now he's all over the news and everyone says, "This is the biggest breakthrough in depression today!" He proved people who have two incomes are less likely to become depressed. People who are financially or not geographically stuck are less likely to get depressed. He proved if your life's good you're not going to become depressed. And he was applauded, however, when I said the same thing. I was the enemy. I'm anti-hero.

In many ways, "depression" is an easy way to absolve responsibility. "I'm fat." "My life's shit." "I'm depressed." Look, depression is a result of your life choices. Your life choices are not a result of your depression. You've got it the wrong way around. And it's just another excuse people use—people need excuses. They don't want to take a cold hard look in the mirror and say, "I'm weak" or "I'm lazy." Instead, they want to say, "I'm depressed." Now, I'm not saying it's impossible to feel depressed. But what I am saying is change your situation and you won't feel depressed. It's that simple, and it comes down to choice.

**Daniel Kelly:** Today weakness is almost seen as a virtue, and qualities such as physical and mental strength are shunned. Why do you think this is?

**Andrew Tate:** People always insult qualities they don't have. A weak person isn't going to stand up and say, "You know what, I am weak, and being strong is really important." Instead, what they say is, "It's 2018, we're not cavemen! And what do you need muscles for? Why do you need to go to the gym? You're just a meathead, moron!" They'll try to justify their stance, because no one wants to admit their faults. And mental strength is a difficult thing to have. So the world's weaklings, they come up and say, "You should cry all the time! Let your wife tell you what to do!" What a joke. Now think about this example. Imagine you're just about to be born and have the chance to shape your character. NOBODY would choose to be a mentally and physically weak pussy! Everyone would choose to be mentally and physically strong, tall, big—all of these things!

The only way they can change their lives and their body is with hard work, which they don't want to do. So instead of the hard work, they prefer to rationalize their nonsense and attack other people. There's not one of them who wouldn't swap places with a kickboxing world champion. This is a Western phenomenon, man, and has parallels with the fall of Rome. Right now I live in Romania, and they have none of that nonsense here.

When I tell Romanian people about this crap, they say, "What the fuck?" They think I'm lying! Romania suffered communism only 20–30 years ago, so they're thankful for what they've got. And it's a lot more traditional. Women are women, and men are men. Gender roles are clear. It's a completely different atmosphere. Rome didn't fall because they lost one big battle; it slowly eroded because the warrior class of Rome had a comfortable life. They would rather be philosophers or poets and have sex all day, or whatever else they wanted to do. It started to collapse because the men became weak.

There's no way the Western world will continue to run the earth 100 or 200 years from now ... just look at America and Western Europe. Basically, people would rather insult someone's success than work hard and get it themselves. They see a guy with muscles and say, "He's a meathead!" Or maybe he works really hard? "Well, he took steroids!" Maybe he did; maybe he didn't. But even if he took steroids, he still worked hard to get that big. So why the fuck are you sitting there insulting him? Because you're skinny and jealous, that's why.

# EPILOGUE

I want to congratulate you for the investment you made in yourself by reaching the end of this book. If you take the time to implement everything we've discussed in this book, you will become peerless. Why? Because in the words of Henry David Thoreau—most men today lead lives of quiet desperation. Their health in every sense—physical, mental, spiritual, and emotional—is in tatters. As a result, they live a listless existence in a limbo between life and death. They can't think clearly because their minds are shrouded in fog, they can't have sex because they can't get an erection, and they have no energy or passion to follow their dreams. In fact, most men are ready for the graveyard by the time they're 30. You look into their eyes, and the spark that once filled them is no longer present.

I'm not here to say that after you optimize your hormones and take care of your health that you will turn into a rock star overnight. However, one thing I can guarantee you is that you will be able to live your life at the highest possible level. You won't become one of the aforementioned men who aimlessly drift through life, not knowing whether they're alive or dead.

The message in this book is a call to arms. I no longer want you to accept second best in anything you do, and especially when it comes to your health. You and you alone are responsible for your life. And if you want to change it, it starts with your health. It is your duty as a man to be fit and strong. I don't recall any stories about low-energy Vikings or Aztec warriors, do you? Of course not, because they lived life in its fullest expression—true to their masculine nature. Now go forth and conquer.

# THE OPTIMIZED UNDER 35 ACTION PLAN

Now you're ready to change your life and take it to the next level. I've coached countless clients to achieve their health and fitness goals, and I've noticed there are two things that separate those who achieve success from those that don't: accountability and commitment. No matter how disciplined or determined you are, you only have so much willpower. What's more, bad habits are notoriously difficult to break. Therefore, it's important to hold yourself accountable to the goals you set—otherwise they are merely empty promises. And I ask my clients to update me regularly so I can hold them accountable.

Taking action without commitment is an exercise in futility. Because when things get difficult, you'll fold like a house of cards. Commitment gives you the strength and courage to see things through no matter what. I ask my clients to make a commitment to themselves, typically by writing it down on paper. Writing things down helps cement them in your mind—something intangible suddenly becomes very concrete. To this end, I've come up with an action plan for you to follow to help you stay accountable and committed to everything you've learned in this book. You don't HAVE to do anything on this list. Ultimately, it's up to you. But if you do follow this plan, I'm confident you'll see incredible results.

1) Write down a summary of the five key lessons you've learned from this book. It can be as long or short as you want.

2) How committed are you to improving your health and fitness? Write down this commitment to yourself and put it somewhere you'll see it regularly (e.g., in your bathroom when you brush your teeth).

3) With regard to your health and fitness goals, what exactly do you want to achieve? Be specific, and put a deadline on it. For example, I want to lose 10 lbs six months from now. Is your

goal realistic, or is it wishful thinking? Most people fail to achieve their health and fitness goals because they're totally unrealistic. You want to get the balance: be realistic while challenging yourself at the same time.

4) What are the steps you're going to have to take to achieve your goals? Perhaps it means you train three times a week, follow a specific diet, or hire a coach.

5) Write down some of the habits that are currently holding you back from achieving your goals. Think about how you could replace them with better habits. Understand, you won't be able to change everything overnight. It's a process, but just writing this down will give you new insights.

6) The old adage is that you are the average of the five people you spend most time with. Consider whether the people you spend most time with are a positive or a negative influence on your health and fitness goals. This doesn't mean you cut ties with everyone around you, but become aware of the effect these people have on you. This may lead you to meet people and strike up new friendships.

7) Remember, you are only ever in competition with yourself. So it doesn't matter where your starting point is in comparison to anyone else. Be kind to yourself and congratulate yourself for having the courage to make positive change because the majority of people are scared to death of change. "A journey of 10,000 miles begins with a single step."

8) Eliminate short-term thinking. See this as a lifestyle and accept you're in it for the long haul. Sometimes it may feel like the results aren't materializing. But when this happens, don't give up. Keep showing up; eventually, incredible things will happen—I promise.

9) Oftentimes we come up with elaborate plans like the one above and convince ourselves we will follow through. And as the saying goes, "The road to hell is paved with good intentions." As human beings, we are naturally lazy because our bodies want to conserve energy. Therefore, to circumvent this instinct you must have skin in the game. For example, buying some new gym shoes or placing a bet with a friend that you will go to the gym three times a week. It usually works best when money is involved. When you pay, you pay attention.

10) It's easy to get trapped in a self-development cycle where you only focus on improving yourself. But if you're not careful, it can become an endless void that's never filled. Reading, lifting, etc. are great, but don't forget to smell the roses and enjoy life for what it is. You only get one shot at life, so you may as well make the most of it. Give yourself permission to relax from time to time, and take a break from focusing on your health and self-improvement.

# THANK YOU

Chomping at the bit for more?

Sign up to my mailing list to be notified first of pending book releases and more content on optimizing your health.

What are you waiting for?

Sign up now: www.optimizedarmy.com/signup

After reading the book and putting its ideas into practice, I want you to reach out to me and tell me about your success.

You can connect with me on twitter at @DanielKellyTRT and on my website: www.optimizedarmy.com/contact

Thank you so much for choosing to be on this journey with me—I am honored to share it with you.

Thanks again,

–Daniel Kelly

# A QUICK FAVOR PLEASE?

Before you go, can I ask you for a quick favor?

Thanks, I knew I could count on you.

Would you please leave a review for this book on Amazon?

Reviews are critical for authors—especially self-published ones like me—as it will help me reach more people.

This way I can carry on writing more books to impact your life in a meaningful way.

So please take just a minute to go to Amazon and leave an honest review for this book. I promise it won't take long and I'll be eternally grateful.

I hope you enjoyed reading this book as much as I enjoyed creating it.

–Daniel Kelly

# ABOUT THE AUTHOR

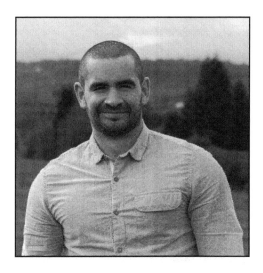

Daniel Kelly is a health and fitness coach, writer and entrepreneur who is extremely passionate about men's health. He aims to help men become the best version of themselves through increasing awareness about their own physical, mental, emotional and spiritual health.

Daniel is a leading authority for men on testosterone replacement therapy, functional health, training and mindset. He strongly advocates that men take responsibility for their health and life, because no one will do it for them. He is a keen traveler and speaks several languages, including French, Spanish, German and Italian. You can find him at optimizedarmy.com and on Twitter @DanielKellyTRT.

Printed in Poland
by Amazon Fulfillment
Poland Sp. z o.o., Wrocław

54412657R00172